Reading Body Language

Everything You Should Know about Body Language to Find out What Every Body is Saying and Foresee Human Behavior and Persuasion

Michael Leary & Gillian Edward

Table of Contents

Introduction 6

Chapter 1: Developing People-Reading Skills 12

Why You Need To Develop Your People-Reading Skills 13

People-Reading Skills 17

Chapter 2: Body Language – The Basics 36

The Science behind Body Language 37

Rules of Reading Body Language 39

Myths about Body Language 42

Chapter 3: Reading Body Parts 48

Chapter 4: Facts about Male and Female Body Languages 72

Men and Body Language Facts 75

Women and Body Language Facts 82

Chapter 5: What A Handshake Says 89

The Importance of a Handshake 90

Types of Handshakes and Their Meanings 93

Giving a Proper Handshake 102

Tips and Tricks about Handshakes 105

Chapter 6: The Language of the Eyes 111

Tips on Initiating Eye Contact 112

Eye Movements and Possible Indications 116

Different Settings, Different Eye Contact 123

Chapter 7: Rapport Building Techniques **128**

Using The Chameleon Effect to Quickly Build Rapport 130

Rapport Building Tips to Remember 136

Chapter 8: Attraction Body Language **144**

How to Make a Man Like You 145

How to Make a Woman Like You 150

Chapter 9: Reading Advanced Body Language **155**

Increased Legs and Feet Movement 157

Sitting Face-to-Face 159

Uncrossing Arms and Legs 160

Stealing a Quick Glance at the Time.. 161

Smiling 163

The Battle Stance and Chin Jut 166

Chapter 10: Faking Your Body Language **168**

How to Fake Body Language Effectively....................................... 171

How to Properly Fake Interest in Others...................................... 174

How to Make Others Feel Comfortable Around You 178

How to Fake Self-Confidence 186

Conclusion... **191**

Introduction

Body language and non-verbal cues are as old as verbal communication. In fact, with humans, non-verbal communication usually precedes verbal communication, as infants do not speak words but can communicate with parents effectively. However, many of us tend to place so much attention on developing verbal communication that we forget or ignore the very important role non-verbal cues play in effective communication.

In our daily interactions, we hear what people say and then react to their words. Sometimes, if we are lucky, our reactions or responses are in tune with what they mean. At other times, our reactions to the words we heard them say are very far removed from their intention; this is how misunderstanding creep into our relationships.

It is the general lack of attention to body language that has caused many of our personal and professional relationships to suffer from misunderstandings, heartaches, harsh judgments, and unnecessary conflicts, all of which can be avoided if we know how to pay attention to the body language of those who are around us.

Thankfully, you can begin right now to take advantage of the growing body of knowledge in the area of non-verbal cues and start to improve the quality of your relationships. This knowledge is not reserved only for a few select elites who have somehow managed to study, research, and discover some "dark secret" on how to read people's minds. Instead, this knowledge is simple and readily available to anyone who wishes to explore the deeper meanings of human intentions using body language. As a matter of fact, almost everyone uses this knowledge to some degree, even though many people do not realize it.

Although this knowledge may be simple, its effect is far-reaching. What you will gain from this book is capable of transforming the way you see and relate to other people - forever! The various facial expressions, head, eyes, and hand movements you had once taken for granted will all take on new meanings. As a matter of fact, you will begin to understand why some of your past personal and professional relationships had issues. You will come to understand that every person you interact with is telling you more than what their words say.

I do not promise that you will become so good at reading body language that you can pass for a mind reader. My promise, however, is that you will clearly understand the fundamental rules that are applicable to reading body language, improve your people-reading abilities, and, to a large extent, determine what other people around you are not saying with their words but which you can clearly perceive. I am giving you the chance to go behind the scenes of people's verbal communication to actually decode what their intentions are.

Equally, this book will expose you to a lot of tricks and tips that you can use to deliberately pass on non-verbal messages to positively influence people for a win-win outcome. I do not offer any form of dark psychology in this book. What I present to you are simple, clear-cut, positive techniques for improving the quality of your interactions with other people, especially those who are important to you.

Beyond the usual information about gestures and their meanings, this book will show you why giving rigid meanings to specific gestures can lead to misunderstandings and errors in judgment. There is no stereotyping when it comes to something as complex as body language. The reason why body language is complex is that there are several factors that can influence people in the way they offer their non-verbal communication.

I wrote this book:

- For the man or woman who want to understand what their partner is saying using their unique body language.

- For the couple who are at the brink of a breakup due to a breakdown of effective communication.

- For the employer who wants to be on the same page with his or her employees.

- For the entrepreneur who is trying to figure out who their next business partner is.

- For the salesperson who wants to clearly sense

objections from a mile away and get into the minds of his or her clients.

- For the parent who really wants to connect with their children on a deeper level.

- For the teacher who loves to help their students seek out their future.

- And for the counselor/therapist who intends to be more helpful to their clients and patients.

I urge you to take all the time you need to diligently study this book. You will be absolutely pleased by the depth of rich information you will be exposed to and the practical ways to apply them in your daily life.

Chapter 1: Developing People-Reading Skills

We lie a lot! Human words are designed to hide true emotions and feelings, making it possible to say one thing and mean the exact opposite. It is not uncommon for people to lie with their words more than once within a conversation that lasts for only about 30 minutes. However, within this same period, our bodies have a way of saying precisely what we are trying so hard to hide. In order to connect with the truest intentions of people, it is necessary to go beyond mere words to actually dig up what their words are not saying.

Why You Need To Develop Your People-Reading Skills

Why go through the stress of learning how to read subtle non-verbal messages when you can simply rely on people's words? Can't we just take people by their word? Must we all become detectives in order to communicate with our friends, families, colleagues, and even strangers? Is it ethical to try to influence people with our body language? Is it right to give meaning to other people's body language? Are we not putting ourselves in a position to misconstrue other people's innocent body movement and gestures?

Well, there are tons of questions that can arise from the subject of body language reading, but the fact remains that we cannot communicate effectively using only words. In the next chapter, when we look at the science behind body language, you'll get to discover that communication even between lower animals can be very effective without words. But for now, let me quickly summarize some of the key reasons why you need to be giving serious thought to developing your people-reading skills.

1. Developing the skills necessary to read people like an open book will help you navigate your social and professional life quite easily.

2. You will be able to hear the words that people say and quickly juxtapose them with what they are not saying so that you can reach a more informed conclusion.

3. You can predict people with some degree of accuracy so long as you take some key factors into consideration.

4. Your relationships (professional and social) are

likely to get better because you can understand people better and therefore connect with them on a deeper level.

5. You reduce unnecessary misunderstandings and heartaches because you can see what others are "saying" that is not meant for the ears to hear no matter how loud the "volume" of the communication is.

6. If you are in a situation that can cause you any harm or hurt in some way, you can learn about this early enough, even when no one is verbally suggesting that you may be hurt.

7. Your people-reading skills are as important as how good you are at your job if you want to improve the quality of your work. The better you get at reading people, the easier it is to sell your ideas, services, and products to your prospects, clients, employers, or colleagues.

8. Reading non-verbal cues is essential for developing Emotional Intelligence, an essential tool for relating well with people at work and at

home.

9. Building your relationships based on mere words is limiting yourself to the superficial aspects of other people. At best, that is a shallow relationship.

A Quick Word of Caution

Keep in mind that the purpose of learning how to read body language is to understand other people better. If you already have a preconceived notion about a person, it can cloud your judgment as you try to assign meaning to what their non-verbal cues are saying.

I would strongly suggest that you keep an open mind when using your people-reading skills to sort through your daily interactions with others. Improving your social and professional relationships should be your main goal for learning how to decode the silent messages that our bodies send.

Now, let's see the exact steps you need to take to develop your people-reading skills.

People-Reading Skills

Understanding what others are saying is quite easy - that is, assuming you know the language being used. Understanding body language, however, is not that easy. Here's why:

- Body language does not mean the same thing 100% of the time.

- Some people are very good at hiding their non-verbal cues.

- Body language is sometimes very subtle and can quickly pass unnoticed.

Generally speaking, reading people's body language means looking for mostly involuntary body movements such as hand gestures, facial expressions, fidgeting, and so on. There are other body languages that are voluntary, such as when someone is trying to communicate discreetly. In any case, when you are trying to read people and analyze their body language, ask yourself:

- What does their posture say?

- Do they appear comfortable or tensed up?

- Are they shuffling their legs, crossing them, or gently hitting them against a chair leg?

- Are they on the edge of their seat?

- Do they suddenly pause or stop talking completely when someone comes nearby?

- Are they talking excitedly, in hushed tones, or with lots of hand gestures?

- Are they leaning toward or away from you (or other people)?

All of these clues and many more give you insight into the true meaning and intentions of the people you interact with. Words alone do not convey these meanings, therefore you must look beyond the surface to decode the meanings.

For you to successfully develop your people-reading skills, you need to understand and keep the following important facts in mind.

Meet With People Face-to-Face

Some decades ago, it was difficult to find one person with thousands of friends. Today, technology has made it very easy to have hundreds of thousands of people in your social circle. You can even make friends and chat with them for several hours without leaving the comfort of your bed. The irony of it is that while making friends is now a lot easier and faster, we have lost the kind of personal touch we use to have when our circle of friends and contacts was a lot smaller.

It is a lot easier to become a communications expert when it is not done face-to-face. These days you will find a lot of people who are really good at communicating via text messages, phones, emails, and so on, but when it comes to face-to-face communication, they take a back seat. Technology has made it possible to communicate with others without necessarily being in the same physical location. This has gradually eroded our people-reading skills. So, rather than walking up to your next door neighbor and having a face-to-face conversation, most people will prefer to simply text or call them. As convenient as this may be, it robs you of a very vital part of communication: the ability to read the other person's non-verbal messages. Have you wondered why people easily argue and fight over comments on social media? One of the reasons is because you cannot accurately gauge a person's true intent by merely reading their comments; you need to see their facial expressions, hear their voice tone, and observe other non-verbal cues in order to properly determine what it is they mean by their words.

I am not in any way against using technology to communicate. However, if you must develop your people-reading skills, then you need to engage more in face-to-face communication. It offers you the chance to actually measure the bodily reactions of the other person and compare them with the tone of their voice before reaching any conclusion. For example, you ask someone out on a date while sitting across from them. Here are some possible responses they could give:

- "No" and from their face and tone of voice, you can tell that they mean no.

- "No," but from the expression on their face, you can tell that they actually don't mean no.

- "Yes" and from the happy look on their face and the inflection of their voice, you can easily tell that they really mean yes.

- "Yes," but from the way they said it, you can tell

that something is off about their agreement.

- "No" but from their facial expression and how their voice sounded, you can tell that they really wish they could say yes.

However, if you ask the same person out using other channels like texting, the response you will get is divorced of all the other vital cues that can give you insight into the emotion behind the response, and you will miss out on all the nuances that may convey a different meaning than what their words say.

So, developing your people-reading skills requires that you, first of all, get back in touch with real humans. Clicking a button on social media that says you like someone doesn't make you a communications expert. If you like someone, walk up to them and tell them so. Walk up to people and give them a warm smile and a sincere compliment. Cultivate the habit of chatting up people in real life even if they are total strangers. Consider the possibility of increasing the frequency of meeting and talking face-to-face with the people you work with or live with instead of texting or phoning them when they are just a few feet away from you. The more you are able to interact with real human beings on a face-to-face basis, the better you will get at improving your people-reading skills.

Careful Observation

Gestures don't always mean the same thing all of the time even for one person. For example, a wink from a trusted friend could be a sign of encouragement, like *"Keep going, you're doing great!"* In another context, that same wink could be a sign to not divulge information, like *"Hush! Don't tell them anything."* Yet, in another situation, it could be a sign of attraction, like *"I can't wait to be with you!"* These are all possible meanings to just one facial gesture.

Body language is not like words written on the pages of a book which usually have the same meaning. The context within which the body language is used is very crucial to the meaning which that non-verbal cue could hold. This is why you need to carefully observe the context or the situation where body language is used before you can come close to understanding its rightful meaning.

This means that part of what you need to learn as you develop your people-reading skills is to take note of the events surrounding the non-verbal cue. What leads up to the interaction where you observed the non-verbal cue is important because that is the context or situation which determines, to a large extent, the silent messages they are sending.

So, in a relaxed environment like a social setting, one gesture could mean a completely different thing than what it would mean in an official or professional setting. If you ignore this and go ahead to give the same meaning to a particular gesture regardless of the context where it is used, you are bound to create miscommunication and misunderstanding with the people you relate with on a daily basis.

Another important thing to remember is that you have to understand a person's general body pattern (or base behavior) before you can accurately read their body language. This means that you need to observe if the other person normally:

- Squints their eyes even when they are

concentrating, listening attentively, or trying to figure things out. Do the same eye movement even when they are just relaxing?

- Drums their fingers when bored or when excited.

- Shifts their weight around in their chair or sits calmly no matter the situation.

- Shifts their weight between their feet when standing for a long time or does the same movement when anxious.

- Spreads their feet apart while firmly planted on the ground when they are angry or in an assertive mood, or stands that way as their usual standing posture.

There are several other body language cues that could mean one thing for someone and yet be just a normal behavior with practically no meaning for another person. When you can determine (to a fair extent) a person's baseline behavior, then you can quickly tell when they have deviated from that behavior and accurately tell that they are silently saying something with their body movements. So, don't rush into trying to give meaning to every single gesture or body movement you notice. First make contact with people, and then take the time to observe and determine what their baseline body pattern is. After that, you can accurately tell what their body language is saying.

This does not mean you cannot read the body language of a complete stranger you just met. However, what it does mean is that you cannot be completely sure of your reading if you do not know the person's baseline behavior. You could be making an intelligent guess, but that could leave room for a wide margin of error.

Be Readable To Some Extent

When people find it difficult to read your intentions, they cannot easily bond with you. The art of reading people is a two-way street that follows the principle of "give and take." If you must build a strong rapport with other people, you need to open up and let them see beyond the words you speak. People are most likely to keep their guard up if they cannot tell which way you lean during an interaction. So, to get past their guard, you need to meet them halfway.

Understand that learning how to read people in the context of this book is not just about being a private detective of some sort. My goal is to show you how to effectively read other people's body language so that you can improve your relationship with them. Therefore, you need to be forthcoming both verbally and non-verbally. If you do not know how to make your body language say exactly what you mean, I strongly suggest that you practice the tips and tricks in the final chapter until you get used to them.

When I say open up or let down your guard, I do not mean that you should throw away your views if they contradict with the views of those who are important to you. Trying to be politically correct all the time will only send the wrong signal to the people in your life. They will view you as someone who is insincere or not authentic. You need to be honest about your views irrespective of whether or not they are acceptable to others. However, if you follow this book to the end, you will discover how to warm your way to other people with your body language, even when you do not necessarily agree with them.

Determine Exactly What You Want in a Relationship

Your personal and professional relationships have to be clearly defined by you. That is to say, you need to determine what it is you would like to experience in each of your relationships.

- What type of friend, partner, or lover are you looking for? What qualities must they possess?

- What kind of business partner are you on the lookout for? What qualifies a person to be the perfect employee that you are looking for?

- What company or organization has the right type of ideas, ideals, and philosophies that you would like to stand with and work for?

It is only when you have clearly defined what you are looking for in your different relationships that your people-reading skills can have any meaningful impact on your life. Think about it for a minute: what will be the benefit of knowing how to read body language and even becoming an expert in it when your relationships with your colleagues, bosses, family, and friends are all in shambles? Prying into other people's true motives and intentions is of little benefit if it does not build you up in any way!

Keep Your Focus on Objectivity

Staying objective when reading people can be a very difficult thing to do, especially if we have vested interest in the person or people we are trying to read. Here are two examples to stress the point I'm trying to make.

John is sexually interested in Kate, his secretary. She has recently not been taking her work seriously and it is beginning to affect the quality of her job. John is finding it difficult to objectively analyze her attitude with respect to her job because of his interest in her. He always finds a way to excuse her obvious body language of disinterest in her job.

John has a new secretary who is not performing her job as expected. John has given her repeated warnings but he can clearly see from her attitude that she is not ready to make corrections. John has no qualms in firing her and looking for a replacement.

Have you ever wondered why no judge is permitted to preside over his or her own case or any case for which it is determined that he or she has vested interest? It is not just because of the Latin phrase *"Nemo judex in causa sua"* (a natural justice principle which means *"no one should be a judge in his own case"*), rather, it is because of bias.

When you have an interest in someone, it is difficult to remain objective, like John in the first example. So, while you are learning to develop your people-reading skills, you must keep your focus on your objectivity, like John in the second example. Keep in mind that emotional attachments are likely to thwart your ability to read people objectively.

Wipe The Slate Clean!

For you to come close to an accurate reading when dealing with people, you must be willing to set aside every previously held prejudice and notions about them. Clear your mind of all preconceived ideas about people of a certain age, sex, race, financial status, and so on. You need to start anew and assess or measure every body movement based on the particular individual and the context in which it occurs, or else you will find yourself erroneously stereotyping people in the false belief that you are reading them. That is a recipe for a completely disastrous relationship!

I strongly suggest that you begin right now to admit your prejudices and then go ahead to let go of them. That is the process of wiping your slate clean so that you can start afresh to assess and evaluate what others are not saying with their words but screaming with their body language.

Decide and Take Action

Do you want to read people's body language effectively? That's awesome! But to what end? If you have taken it upon yourself to meet people face-to-face (even when it is very uncomfortable for you at first), then gone ahead to observe them patiently to determine their baseline behavior so that you can accurately tell when they have deviated from that normal behavior, and then you do nothing with the result of your people-reading ability, what then is the point of following all the processes?

What I am driving at is simple: develop your people-reading skills, go ahead and read people, and then make informed decisions based on your readings. That is to say, if you have determined that a person is cunning or dishonest, take the necessary steps to limit your relationship with that person. On the other hand, if you have assessed a person and found both from their words and body language that they are trustworthy and reliable, then go ahead and strengthen your relationship with them.

Now that we have seen the steps necessary to improve your people-reading skills, let us take a quick look at the very basics of body language.

Chapter 2: Body Language – The Basics

Body language, also known as non-verbal cues, is the conscious and unconscious movements of various parts of the human body that convey the feelings, intentions, and attitudes of an individual. Ordinarily, we should say what we mean, but when our words run contrary to our true intentions, it is very possible that one or more parts of our body will reveal our intention. Equally, we can deliberately or consciously allow our body to buttress and confirm what our words are saying. When you understand how body language works, connecting with others on a deeper level will become easy for you because you know their intentions and how they feel during the period of your interaction with them.

In this chapter, we shall take a look at common body language cues and what they signify. But before we go into that, let us examine the science behind body language very briefly.

The Science behind Body Language

Animals don't talk; that's no news. However, they do communicate in such a distinct manner that misunderstandings are minimized. This goes to show that communication is not only done through words. Humans have the added advantage of communicating using words, but many of us have come to be so used to words that we have forgotten how to deliberately communicate through other means.

It is quite difficult to separate verbal communication from non-verbal communication; the two go hand-in-hand. But while it is a lot easier to communicate verbally, non-verbal communication is a bit more complex than its verbal counterpart. Nevertheless, we are hard-wired to naturally read the emotions of other people and the meaning such emotions hold; this is as a result of mirror neurons inside of our brain that are activated when our mind observes an emotion in another person.

We all possess a conscious and unconscious mind. Additionally, we have our instinct, which is a mind of its own located in our gut (also referred to as the solar plexus). The gut contains as many neurons as the brain in your head, and they are all intricately linked to your unconscious mind. The unconscious mind and your gut are continuously scanning your environment to pick up the emotional states and intentions of the people around you. So, while your conscious mind is busy listening to the words being spoken, your gut and unconscious mind (which are faster at perceiving even the slightest changes in emotional intent) are on the lookout for the intent behind the spoken words you hear. When there is a discrepancy between the words and the unspoken emotional intent, you feel it in your gut – you just know deep down in your stomach that something is not right.

Your job is to deliberately engage your gut and the unconscious mind by practicing the tips and techniques outlined in this book. The more you deliberately engage in this, the better your conscious mind will get at quickly receiving and decoding the message from your gut and unconscious mind.

Rules of Reading Body Language

Briefly, here are 3 very important rules you must remember if you want to properly and accurately read body language.

1. **A cluster of non-verbal cues gives the most accurate reading**. It is easier to make proper sense of a word if you look at it in a phrase or a sentence. The same is true of body language. If you try to read body language in isolation, it may not make sense or it may give you a completely different meaning. The best way to approach reading people is to take a cluster of non-verbal cues into consideration so that you can arrive at an informed conclusion.

Do not base your conclusions on one random body language cue. For example, you may see someone biting their nails and jump to the hurried conclusion that they are nervous, anxious, or afraid of something or someone. However, if you do not take the time to also observe that they have been calmly lying on their couch all day, you may miss the telltale sign that biting their nails is a habit they engage in when they are feeling bored.

2. **Environment and culture matter**. Gestures do not have a universally accepted meaning. This means that one body language cue may indicate a completely different (and sometimes opposite) meaning in one culture and region than it signifies in another culture and region. For example, a nod means an agreement in many cultures, but in places like Japan, it simply means that your listener heard what you said without necessarily agreeing to it. If you were to nod your head in Macedonia as a way of saying "yes," a native will read it as a "no." Men

holding hands in public may be read as a sign that they are homosexual, but in Saudi Arabia, it indicates kinship and solidarity. Giving a thumbs up can easily be read as "good" or "OK," but it may surprise you to learn that it means man in Japan. And here's something that may surprise you further: the reaction of women when they are seen naked varies from place to place. An American or British woman will cover her breast with one hand and use the other hand to cover her genitals. A woman from the Middle East will simply use both hands to cover her face. A Sumatran woman caught naked will quickly cover her knees. If she is from Sweden, her first reaction would be to cover her genitals only. And a woman from Samoan? She will simply cover her navel if caught naked. I am sure you can now see how culture and environment play a major role in body language interpretations. So, be mindful of the background of a person if you must accurately read their body language.

3. **Keep the context in perspective**. As I have mentioned earlier in the previous chapter, body language can mean several things when used in different circumstances. Make sure that you pay attention to the context where particular body language is used before you decode what the body language indicates. So, if you happen to lock eyes with someone of the opposite sex who is licking their lips in a restaurant, for example, it may not automatically mean that they are flirting with you. It could be that they just finished eating or tasted something nice. However, in a club, licking of the lips could take on an entirely different meaning.

Myths about Body Language

1. **Non-verbal cues have universal meanings**. It is easy for people to slip into thinking that a specific gesture, facial expression, and other body language cues have fixed meanings. It is true that some handful of gestures (such as the OK sign, peace sign,

middle finger, and a few others) convey a generally accepted meaning in almost every part of the world. However, it is erroneous to assign specific meanings to all non-verbal cues, because each of us has different ways in which we show our emotional intent. Our body language is influenced by our personality type, environment, and other factors that make it difficult to pin one meaning to specific body language for everybody.

What this means is that when you observe someone scratching the side of their face, for example, it doesn't automatically translate to mean that they are trying to lie. They may simply have an itch! In as much as crossing the arms can mean that a person is defensive, it can also mean that the person is simply cold or they are feeling self-confident. This is why it is a good idea to first establish baseline behavior for a person, as I have earlier mentioned in the previous chapter.

2. **Body language shows exact meaning**.

Another myth about body language is that it conveys an exact meaning. If X behaves in Y manner, it means Z. This is thinking in absolute terms and is likely to result in misunderstandings. What you should always keep in mind is that body language is not a perfect science. While you can know someone's intention from their body language, it is quite difficult to pin it to a definite meaning. For example, it may be safe to say that a woman who looks at a man with the "come hither" look is flirting with him. But to say that she wants to marry him or she wants to have sex with him may not be a correct assumption. Flirting does not always necessarily end in sex or marriage. It could be that she is simply trying to tease him and nothing more. This is where understanding the context within which body language is used comes into play.

To be on the safe side, always remember that body language simply signifies a person's emotional intent. This will help you form a general idea about what they are not saying but what their body language is revealing. Understand that the art of reading body language does not in any way make you know the exact thoughts in people's heads.

3. **You must be an expert to accurately read people**. While I do not wish to discount the need to become a psychology expert or to belittle the work which experts in the field put into body language research, the truth is that you don't have to necessarily try too hard before you can know how to read people, especially those who are currently in your life.

If you have spent quite some time with the current people at work, home, school, or any other place, chances are that you already know their baseline behaviors. This means you can tell when they are not happy (even when they try to hide it) and you can also tell when they are happy. You can tell when their words are not in sync with their body language. These things do not require you to become an expert at body language reading.

4. **The face shows our true intentions**. This myth is deeply rooted in the false premise that our whole lives show in our faces. While it is true that your face has the capacity to show a lot of emotions (21 different emotions!), most adults are adept at masking their emotions and effectively keeping them from showing up on their faces. The need to get along with others, avoid conflicts, and be socially acceptable drives us to pretend and keep our true emotional intent away from our faces. However, this pretense is usually a form of polite deception; it is not usually aimed at hurting other people.

The fact is that our faces do show micro-expressions which are difficult to mask. But do not depend solely on people's facial expressions to let you into their true intentions. Other parts of the body show people's true intentions much more clearly than their faces.

Chapter 3: Reading Body Parts

There is no part of the human body that is redundant when it comes to conveying unspoken intentions. From the crown of our heads down to the tips of our toes, every part of the body plays some role in communication. Even our skin can reveal a lot about how we feel; it can become flushed and can also instantly generate goosebumps to communicate how we are feeling in a particular moment.

Although "talking" with our body parts may not be audible, others around us can pick up the messages loud and clear, especially if they are versed in the art of reading people. Keep in mind that people, adults especially, usually are good at hiding their feelings and intentions from showing up on their faces, so they may want to cover up their body language with polite facial expressions and words. However, if you are observant enough, you can pick up discrepancies between their words and other parts of the body that are a bit difficult to consciously manipulate.

The good news is that since not many people go through training to hide or fake their body language, they usually don't keep up the act for long. This means, if you take the time to study people, you will get to know when they are putting up appearances and when they are being real.

Here are some of the cues from different parts of the body and the likely intention that they signify.

The Head

Head movements can be quite easy to read if you know how to. Unfortunately, not everyone knows how to do this, which is why even the most obvious head movements go unnoticed by the ignorant and inexperienced person.

Let us assume you are a salesperson delivering your well-practiced sales pitch to a prospective client. The potential buyer appears engrossed in the sales pitch but at a point, he tilts his head slightly back. If you do not understand this subtle head movement, you will carry on with your sales pitch without pausing to ask if the potential buyer or client want something you said clarified. Your sales pitch is important, but it will be ineffective if you cannot quickly identify silent objection signals.

Here's another example of a head movement. Your junior colleague is nodding at almost everything you said during a practice presentation. You assume that he is showing his agreement, understanding, or confirming what you are saying to be correct. Unknown to you, he is merely being polite and hiding his urge to scream, *"Get it over with already, will you!"* Ignorantly, you have failed to note that nodding could be a sign of disinterest. It could also be that they are simply agreeing with your ideas as a form of lip service so that they can be in your good books.

Let us take a look at the most common head movements alongside what they may be possibly indicating.

- Let's start with a nod. In most parts of the world, a nod indicates encouragement. However, not all nods are made equally. When a person nods slowly, especially if they are doing it unconsciously, it connotes a deep level of interest or rapt attention. Another head movement that indicates interest is when the person tilts their head sideways. So, if you are making some form of presentation in class or at a meeting and you notice these two head movements, it is very likely that your points are well expressed and understood.

- Hurried nods or frequent nods during a presentation could signal disinterest like in the second example above. If you notice this during your presentation or discussion, change your tactics or presentation style. Alternatively, pause the presentation and ask for input from the other person or people.

- In the case where a person tilts their head back while you are talking with them, it is a possible sign of disbelief, doubt, or suspicion. Whether it is a one-on-one conversation or a formal presentation in front of a board of directors, take a moment to clarify what you were talking about before you noticed that head movement. If you are unsure, ask them if there is something they would like you to make clearer. You could say, *"I'm getting the feeling that you may need some further clarifications. Would you like me to clarify my last point or something I've said earlier?"*

- When talking with a friend and they begin to scratch an imaginary itch on their necks or the side of their face or their jaw, this is usually body language of disagreement. Give the other person room to speak their mind by saying something along the lines of, *"It looks like you have something different in mind. What is it?"* This can also happen when you are speaking in a formal meeting. In the event that you are leading the discussions or in the case where it is appropriate for that particular meeting, you can give the person with the disagreeing body language a chance to say what's on their mind. You could say, *"I see Mr. X has something to say. Would you please give us your point of view on this?"*

- In an official meeting, head movements can tell you who is in charge or who wields more authority. In a meeting, most heads will be turned towards the person who has the most authority.

- The use of head movement is not limited to only formal meetings and during chitchats with friends. It can also speak volumes even in situations that do not require discussions. When someone stands with their head held upwards, it can signify arrogance, self-confidence, or superiority. This is especially true if their chin points forward.

- Head held downwards could indicate a negative attitude or aggression. Subconsciously, our minds know that our intentions are not pure. Therefore it makes us unconsciously protect our neck and throat, which are vulnerable parts of our body, by lowering our heads to cover them. This is subconscious body language to keep us safe in case the other person attacks us if they get wind of our intentions.

- It is common knowledge that when someone shakes their head from side to side, it indicates rejection, disagreement, denial, or a simple "no" except in places like Bulgaria, Macedonia, and Albania. Nevertheless, the rhythm and speed of a head shake can give it a lot of different meanings depending on the part of the world which you find yourself. When a person shakes their head in a quick rhythmic way, that's a way to say "*I do not agree. This is not true.*" When the pace is slow with an irregular rhythm, that usually is a sign of misunderstanding. The person is silently saying, "*I think something is off.*" A slow head-shake with a regular rhythm is most likely a way of indicating disbelief, especially as a reaction to something we have just recently heard.

- The last head movement I shall discuss is the head bobble. This is usually seen in places like India. It does not indicate a no or a yes. Instead, it can indicate a greeting, "yes," "no," "thank you," and even "maybe" depending on the circumstances in which it is used coupled with very slight alterations that are completely lost on a foreigner. Here's the point of all this: if you happen to visit any foreign country, you can build rapport with the natives by copying their customs and culture. Even if you do not get it perfectly, they will be glad that you respect them and want to learn about them.

The Face

The face conveys messages that are very obvious to notice. Expressions such as frowns, smiles (grin or smirk), grimaces, dropped jaw, squinting, raised eyebrows, yawns and so on can be read by almost everyone. Since it is not difficult to decode the emotional intent (anger, excitement, surprise, fear, confusion, disgust, and so on) by simply looking at the face, most of us have learned how to effectively hide these indicators so that we can appear polite. That notwithstanding, a careful study of a person's face can still reveal true intentions.

The following are some of the facial expressions and what they signify.

- A smile is one body language cue that has a universal meaning. Even infants can read this non-verbal cue. It strongly indicates acceptance, agreement, and comfortableness. When a smile spreads to cover the entire face, it is genuine.

- When a smile doesn't reach the eyes of the giver – when there are no crinkles at the corners of their eyes – it shows that it is a forced or fake smile. There are several reasons a person would want to wear a fake smile. They may want to be polite, they may want to be deceitful, or they simply want to seek approval from another person, especially from someone superior.

- A slight smile accompanied by a slightly raised eyebrow is one facial expression that indicates confidence and friendliness. When you are talking with someone and notice this expression on the person's face, it indicates that they believe what you are saying. If you are the one wearing this expression, you are conveying to the other person that you are trustworthy.

- The lips are used for smiling and also for telling truth or falsehood. When someone touches their lips repeatedly while telling you something supposedly confidential, there is a high chance that they are withholding some of the information from you.

The Eyes

There are a whole lot of messages that can be passed using the eyes. I shall mention only a few here. In a subsequent chapter, I'll go into detail about the eyes.

- When someone keeps their eyes looking downward, it is an indication that they are feeling guilt, shame, or they are simply shy. For example, a child who has done wrong and feels guilty will likely keep their eyes down when their parents speak to them about what they've done. Also, a shy person is very likely to look down in the presence of someone they are not used to. When someone feels another person is very superior to them, they will look downward not as a sign of shame, guilt, or shyness, but as an indication of submissiveness. A very junior worker in a company, for example, is most likely to keep their gaze on the floor when they are in the presence of the company's CEO.

- When the person you are conversing with keeps stealing a look at the exit, it is a strong indication that they want to get away from that conversation to something else. It could also indicate that they are nervous, anxious, or apprehensive about something which their words are not saying but their body is communicating very clearly.

- When someone is continuously avoiding eye contact with you, it could indicate several things. One of the possible reasons could be that they are shy. However, if you take other factors into consideration (context and cluster), you should be able to tell whether or not they are truly shy. If they are hurriedly trying to get you to give your consent about something, like signing a deal, and they keep on avoiding your eyes during the interaction, in that context, it has nothing to do with being shy. Instead, it is a strong indication that they are not being completely honest with you. If they only avoid your eyes when you look at them but steal glances at you when they think you are not looking, it could be that they are interested in you or they are flirting with you.

The Shoulders

Shrugging is usually considered as a sign of ignorance or cluelessness. However, it can indicate other things such as an unconscious need to protect our necks (vulnerable part) from danger. For example, notice how people generally react with they hear a sudden loud bang of a gun or even a seemingly harmless thing like a balloon bursting. The first reaction for most people is to raise their shoulders to hide their neck. You can also observe this when people walk in front of a crowd that is focused on something, like a movie in a cinema. The person walking in front of the crowd tends to shrug so that their necks are hidden inside their shoulders in an unconscious attempt to protect themselves in case of an attack from the angry crowd. Even children speak this unconscious protective body language when they hide their necks by raising their shoulders if their parents attempt to hit them.

Hand Movements and Gestures

- Keep your hands out of your pocket if you want to communicate openness and honesty. When you have your hands in your pocket, your body language is saying you don't have self-confidence, you are hiding something, or you are being defensive.

- When someone has their palms facing up as they are talking, that gesture strongly suggests that they are being honest. It does not necessarily mean that their views are correct, but it does show that they are genuinely expressing their thoughts.

- Someone holding an object between you and them is unconsciously trying to put a barrier between you and them. Their body language is indicating that they are looking for any excuse to block you out. For example, if a salesperson is trying to sell a product to a prospective customer, and the customer keeps fidgeting with a book, a paper bag, or just about anything, it will serve the salesperson well to first turn his or her attention to enlisting their trust before attempting to sell them anything.

- When someone habitually points to another person while talking in a group or in a meeting, it is a strong indication that they have many things in common or they have some type of affinity. Here's a great way you can use that to your advantage, especially in a situation where you are canvassing for support: seek the support of one of the pair, and you are most likely to get the support of the other.

The Arms

- When someone has their arms crossed along their chest while beaming with a warm smile, it signifies self-confidence.

- However, the same body pose without the smile is likely to indicate aggression, disagreement, or defensiveness.

- Placing the hands on the hips suggests dominance, power, or authority. This can also take the form of placing the hands firmly on a table while standing behind the table. For example, a boss or superior in an office can take this pose to add emphasis to the point they are making.

The Feet

One of the most ignored body parts when it comes to body language is the feet. Yet, the feet reveal a lot more than people realize. So, while people work so hard to hide their emotional intent from their faces, their feet may be all you need to observe in order to understand what is truly going on inside of them. Here's what to look out for:

- When someone's feet are pointing towards the door when you are talking with them, they are probably thinking about leaving or ending that line of discussion. Take the cue and summarize what you are saying or change the topic completely.

- When the other person's feet are pointing towards you, it signifies that they are interested in you or whatever it is you are saying. It may also indicate that they like you. If you are presenting an idea to a person and notice this signal, cash in on this opportunity to hit hard on your strong points in order to win them over quickly before they get bored and their feet turn towards the door!

- When someone is nervous or feeling apprehensive, they are likely to have their ankles locked. The locked ankles are usually unconsciously used during an uncomfortable discussion. For example, when a friend is talking with you about a not-so-pleasant event in an environment that is not private, they may lock their ankles to signify that they are worried about another friend walking in during the discussion. The ankle lock can also indicate that a person is nervous about some news. For example, a patient waiting for a doctor's report may unconsciously lock their ankles in nervous anticipation of the report. If you notice this body language with someone you are talking with, you can take the cue and try to calm them down if the situation makes it appropriate for you to do that.

Body Mirroring

When you see someone yawning, there is a good chance that you will yawn also. That is a form of unconscious body mirroring. When you deliberately or unconsciously copy someone else's body movement or speech pattern, it is known as body mirroring. It is also referred to as the chameleon effect – taking on the semblance of your immediate environment.

Body mirroring can be a very useful tool if you use it wisely and sparingly. Here are some tips that you should remember when using body mirroring.

- Don't mirror body languages that have negative connotations. For example, if your colleague at work usually clenches and unclenches their fists as their unspoken way of saying they are angry, copying that body language is likely going to make them want to avoid you because they will unconsciously perceive you as a negative or angry person. Here's the thing: negative emotions are unpleasant whether or not it is us who feels them. It doesn't matter if you were only mirroring them; you remind them of emotions they don't like to experience and they will begin to avoid you.

- You can tell if someone is into you by observing if they are unconsciously mirroring your body movements. To confirm this, change your body posture. Do this in a way that is not too obvious that you are monitoring them, and then wait for a few seconds to see whether or not they adjust their posture to suit yours. If they do, you have struck a bond with them at that moment and you can seize the opportunity to sell them your ideas, opinions, or simply build a stronger relationship with them.

- Generally, men consider dressing alike as a sign of friendship. A man can go the extra length of seeking out another man that dresses like him in a crowd to strike a bond of friendship.

- Generally, women do not like other women to dress exactly like them. If you are a woman, it is a gross mistake to think that dressing like another woman will help you to build a strong rapport with her. You can mirror any other thing about her, but not her outfit!

Personal Space

The amount of physical space between people can convey a great deal of non-verbal information the same way facial expressions and body movements can. It can reveal the level of interest a person has in you. Note the following about personal space:

- When someone is comfortable around you, they don't mind sitting or standing very close to you. If you observe this, it is a chance for you to make your relationship even stronger. That is, if you like the person.

- When someone is uncomfortable around you or they do not share a connection with you, they are very likely to sit or stand away from you. If you observe this, it is an opportunity for you to put in more work into that relationship if you really like the person and the relationship is important to you.

But how close is close enough and how far away from you is far enough? Although there is no hard and fast rule about this, here is a general idea to guide you.

- When a person's physical proximity to you is about 18 to 6 inches (15 to 45 cm) or even less, and you are comfortable with that physical closeness, there is a loud and clear non-verbal message that says you share some deep level of intimacy with the person (such as a romantic partner or your spouse) or you are in a very close personal relationship with the person (such as your child, siblings, parent, or very close friends). If a person who does not share a very close connection with you steps into this personal space of yours, it could mean they are a physical threat to you.

- When a person stands or sits at about 18 to 46 inches (45 cm to 1.2 meters) away from you, it indicates that they are friendly with you but not intimate. In social gatherings, you will notice that people usually maintain this distance to allow room for socially acceptable interactions. This is the type of distance that you should keep if you don't want your friend to begin to think you are crowding their personal space. However, if you intend to take your relationship with a friend to another level – from the friend zone to the intimate zone – you should gradually begin to close the gap in this distance in an unobtrusive manner.

- For people who you've just met, like strangers, or for those who are not really your friends but casual acquaintances, a distance of about 4 to 12 feet (1.2 to 3.5 meters) is considered good enough during interactions. When you begin to cross this boundary, you may spook them or make them think you have an ulterior motive. For example, if a man gets too close to a lady who is a total stranger in a deserted alley, she is likely to scream for help or back away and break into a run even if the man meant no harm. His body language led to that misunderstanding and the negative reaction/response.

- A distance of over 12 feet (3.5 meters) is perfectly okay for addressing a group of people in a meeting, class, or any other kind of gathering.

Chapter 4: Facts about Male and Female Body Languages

Although we are all human beings, it is very obvious that men and women are wired and built a bit differently both physically and psychologically. This means that while we may all use non-verbal cues to communicate our true intentions, these intentions or meanings may be slightly different depending on the gender of the person. For example, when a man touches the side of his neck while talking or looking at someone, it could mean a completely different thing than when a woman makes the same body movement. Misconstruing this body language to mean the same thing for genders may lead to inaccurate interpretation of intentions.

Men tend to be more obvious with their non-verbal cues than women. For example, when a man is interested in a woman, he checks her out in an obvious manner. He may even be direct and approach her or engage her in some chit chat with several gestures that clearly say *"I am interested in you!"* On the other hand, a woman is subtler with her body language. If, for example, she is interested in a man, you will hardly catch her checking him out! This is not to say that women don't check men out, but they do it in such a way that affords them the chance to deny it (what is otherwise called plausible deniability).

I have outlined below a few interesting facts about the way men and women communicate non-verbally. Pay particular attention to these differences so that you will not make the mistake of generalizing body languages and their meanings. Note that the purpose of this chapter, and in fact, this book, is to acquaint and equip you with the essential knowledge you need to effectively read non-verbal cues. What this means is that, it doesn't matter if you are a male or female, you can become very good at reading body language and at the same time mask or reveal whatever non-verbal cues you choose. That is to say, if you are a man reading this book, know that although men are generally considered to be slower than women at reading body language, you can learn how and eventually become very good at quickly reading anyone you come in contact with, irrespective of their gender.

Men and Body Language Facts

The Male Brain

From an evolutionary point of view, men have fewer areas activated in their brains when they read a person's body language. Men have only about 4 to 6 brain areas active while they process non-verbal cues; women, on the other hand, have about 14 to 16 different brain areas activated during the same process! This can be clearly seen in an MRI scan. It is no wonder that women tend to be better at reading or evaluating people's behavior than men.

Slower Rate of Decoding Non-Verbal Cues

Following the above fact, men tend to be slower when reading people's body language. This is particularly true when a woman is trying to pass subtle messages to a man, especially messages that indicate that she is interested in him. For example, a woman sitting across from a man can gaze at a man with the intent of letting him know that she wants him, but he just wouldn't notice this gaze. To any other woman observing the subtle interaction, it is a crystal clear message, but the man or other men in the same setting will simply miss it altogether. Research has shown that on average, a woman has to make at least 3 different signals to a man in order to catch his attention (Barker, 2014).

Motive for Lying

No matter the name we call it when our words say differently from what our non-verbal cues are conveying, it simply means at that moment we are lying, period! Men do this (lying) usually for very different purposes than women. For men, the reason for lying, either verbally or nonverbally, is usually to make themselves appear better than they actually are. They want others to perceive them as more successful, interesting, or powerful than they truly are. Another interesting thing about lying for men is that they are likely to lie more about themselves than about others. In order words, the focus for men's lies is to draw attention to themselves.

Attraction Signal

Men have a way with their feet. When it points towards a person it is more than likely that they are attracted to that person or they are very interested in that person. On the flip side, men are likely to have their feet pointing towards the door or the available exit when they are uninterested in the person they are interacting with.

Flirting Signal

Men have their own ways of showing interest (sexually) in other people without verbalizing it. When you notice any of these body language cues, there is a very good chance that the man is sexually interested in you or he may be simply flirting with you.

- When a man leans in closely toward you while speaking or interacting with you.

- When a man's gaze goes from mere glances to intimate gazing. His gaze starts by looking into your eyes and gradually travels down to your mouth, and then down to your neck and the rest of your body. This is a rather clear flirting signal.

- Smiling. This is a difficult body language to interpret if the man with the smile is not really nearby to observe their eyes. It may be difficult to tell if it is a fake or real smile. But regardless of whether is a genuine or fake smile, when a man smiles at someone more frequently than usual, it may mean that they are interested in the person they are smiling at.

- Putting on an expressive face. Men tend to allow their feelings and desire to show on their face when they are interested in the person they are talking to or interacting with. Winks, raised eyebrows, excessive smiling and so on during contact is like letting the face say what the words aren't saying. *"I like you; I hope you can read it on my face!"*

- When a man shows his hands when conversing, it is a sign of interest. When his hands become more animated (not in angry gestures) and hardly stay in his pockets, he may be interested in the other person in more ways than one.

- When a man touches a woman (or another man) on their forearm, face, or on the waist, it can be a serious level of flirting. When the touch is formal, like a handshake or a shoulder tap, it may simply be a friendly touch. But an informal gentle or soft touch that can lead to a hug is more likely to mean a deeper interest in the other person.

What Attracts Men

Men are more attracted by the behavior that says "*I am available*" than they are attracted by good looks. Of course, a good-looking woman has a plus because men are easily moved by what they see. But beyond the first physical attraction, what will make a man really interested and drawn to a woman is a behavior that indicates that she is open. Here's a clear example to drive home the point. Suppose there are two equally attractive women, one with an open attitude and the other with a distant or closed attitude. Who between the two do you suppose the man will be more drawn to? Of course, he'll be easily drawn to the one with an open attitude. That is to say that flirtatious behavior is much more likely to attract a man than a mere pretty face.

Women and Body Language Facts

The Female Intuition

The fact that women are more perceptive or more attuned to their intuitive senses is not a hoax or a mere myth. Scientific evidence reveals that the female brain has increased blood flow compared to that of men (Morad, 2017). In a study which evaluated 46,000 different studies of more than 25,000 male and female adults, scientists also found that the female memory center (hippocampus) is more active than in men (Amen, D. et al., 2017). This means women are more likely to remember details than men.

While non-verbal cues may easily pass unnoticed by men, women are more likely to catch the faintest whiff of any discrepancy existing between words spoken and body language. Most of all, they will remember that detail for a very long time.

Motive for Lying

Women lie (especially non-verbally) for different reasons than men do, and when they do, it is more often about other people than it is about themselves. Here's what I mean by that: it is more likely that a woman's lies are about protecting someone else – to make others feel good about themselves or preserve their dignity. This is why even when it hurts them, women tend to lie to protect those they love.

Submissive Cues

Here are some body language cues that indicate that a woman "wants to be rescued" or is being submissive. Appearing vulnerable is the motive behind these non-verbal cues.

- Exposing the wrists is an unconscious sign of vulnerability. A limp wrist also has the same effect as exposing the wrist. Notice that men who smoke tend to bring the cigarette up to their mouth and back down with the back of their hand showing in one smooth motion, but most women who smoke tend to make the same move with their wrist exposed while taking their hands away from their mouth.

- Putting on a helpless look by plucking the eyebrows higher on the forehead is a perfect way to take advantage of the man's inborn desire to be protective of the woman.

Assertive Cues

When a woman stands with her feet firmly planted on the ground and spread a bit further apart, it is an indication that she is very self-confident. This body language is known as "claiming territory" and I discuss it further in the final chapter.

Flirting Signal

Women have a way of sending subtle messages with their body to indicate sexual interest or something close to that. They can do this consciously, and other times they are not even aware that their body language is screaming what their words are not saying. One reason many women are not overly apparent when flirting is so that they can save face and retain some self-dignity if the person they are flirting with turns out not to be interested in them.

If you are a man, you'll find the following information very useful to note so that you can tell when a woman is telling you that she's into you and decide whether or not to take the cue. If you are a woman, you'll also find this information very useful so that you can attract the man you really want. And if you truly are not interested in a person, you will know how to not send them mixed messages.

- Women flirt with several body movements like playing with their ears, tilting their head and flipping their hair to expose their neck area, slightly biting or licking their lips, showily crossing and uncrossing their legs, or slowly stroking their body.

- Perhaps the most clearly visible body language that a woman is interested in and flirting with you is blushing. When a woman blushes (on the cheeks, upper chest, or lower neck area) because you looked at her or said something to her, she's likely into you. Blushes are uncontrolled and indicate an increase in the heart rate. Sexual excitement is closely linked to this unconscious reaction.

- When a woman keeps "accidentally" bumping into you, especially at a social event, there is a possibility that she's lurking around you and trying to get your attention.

- When women experience pleasure (especially sensual pleasure), one of their common facial expressions is to slightly raise their eyebrows while lowering their eyelids. But this expression is not limited to intimate pleasures alone. When a woman looks at you with that expression on her face, the chances that she's trying to entice you are very high.

- Women can draw a man's attention to their pelvic area by swaying their hips while walking away from or towards the man. When a woman sticks out her hips sideways in a rather provocative way, she is trying to draw attention to her hips.

- Women value their bodily accessories, but when they begin to play with these accessories while interacting with you, it could be that they are showing signs of interest in you. Fiddling with her jacket or shirt button, necklace, earrings, or when she lets her shoe dangle from her toes while she's sitting across from you are clear indications that she feels comfortable with you.

- Giggling at almost every one of your comments or every joke you make (even if they are not funny).

- A woman dancing all by herself at a party is

silently saying *"I am available!"*

- Looking at you long enough to catch your eyes and then looking away quickly when your eyes catch hers.

- When a woman lets her guard down and becomes freer with you such that she whispers in your ear, teases you, or begins to use words that have two meanings with one usually having a sexual connotation (entendre), she is probably interested in you in a sexual or romantic context.

- When a woman consciously or unconsciously runs her hand through her hair while talking with you, it may indicate flirting. She can begin to curl her hair, tuck it behind her ears, twirl it, tie it up and take it down again – all of these are signs of interest.

Chapter 5: What A Handshake Says

In the space of 3 to 6 seconds of making physical contact with a person, you can read a ton of information about their personality even if you are just meeting them for the very first time. A handshake may last for a very brief moment, but it has the capacity to make us look good, bad, confident, insecure, or completely clueless. The first impression, they say, matters a lot. The first physical contact you are most likely to have with anyone is the handshake. If you do not deliver it properly, it paints you in a very different light from who you truly are.

In this chapter, we shall consider all the things that you need to know about this very powerful non-verbal cue so that you will be able to use it to your advantage. At the end of this chapter, you will no longer see a handshake as a mere courtesy tool or a way to greet people. You will see that just as it is important to improve your appearance and voice in order to impress people (especially if you are meeting them for the first time), it is equally important to learn how to give a proper handshake to convey the right type of message you want to send to others.

The Importance of a Handshake

Beyond being a sign of friendliness, courtesy, and greeting, a handshake is capable of:

- Opening doors of great opportunities for business or closing shut the doors of businesses.

- Creating a long-lasting friendship and partnership or halting any chance of a further relationship.

- Telling others who you are.

The truth is that the impression created by your handshake goes way beyond the brief seconds that the handshake lasted. In a business setting, everything you have so carefully prepared could come crashing down by your first handshake. Therefore, you need to be sure of what your handshake says about you. In a social setting, handshakes can be used as a polite way of initiating physical contact with another person. For example, you can seize the opportunity of a handshake to touch someone you are attracted to and send them non-verbal messages to indicate your interest in them.

Equally, there are several types of handshakes (high five, fist bump, and so on) that are meant for different settings and occasions. If you use a handshake meant for social settings during a business meeting, for example, you may completely ruin your chances of closing any deal. Another example would be to give a handshake that says you are submissive when the message you really want to convey is that you are in charge.

There may be no school where handshakes are taught, but thankfully, you have access to this book where you can begin to learn how to convey the correct message using this body language. Now let's see the different types of handshakes and the exact messages they convey.

Types of Handshakes and Their Meanings

Handshakes have evolved over the years and are still evolving. Different groups can decide what modification to adopt and what meaning to assign to it. But we shall only concern ourselves with the generally known types and see what they mean.

Standard Handshake

First, I'll start with the standard handshake. What I mean by a standard handshake is that it can be used for both professional and social settings without making you look out of place. However, you will want to play it down a bit when using this type of handshake in a social setting where the people you are meeting are very close to you so that your body language won't convey an uptight message to them.

To give the Standard Handshake, ensure that your grasp is firm, hand is dry, and that your palm goes into the other person's palm in a sideways, web-to-web fashion. Make sure that your fingers are stretched out straight in front of you and your thumb is facing up. Wear a warm smile and lock eyes with the receiver of your handshake.

Bone Crusher

Bone Crusher is used to display intimidation. The giver puts on an extra squeeze as if crushing the receiver's hand. This type of handshake has an emotional bully written all over it. Avoid it by all means, unless of course you want to be seen by the receiver as an aggressive person. Keep your handshake firm but do not crush the other person's hand to show superiority. That will only worsen your relationship with them.

Dead Fish

One of the worst types of handshake you could ever give is the dead fish (or limp fish). There is practically no life in this type of handshake – it is cold, devoid of energy, vigor, and without any form of squeeze whatsoever! It is like grabbing a dead, slippery fish; no one enjoys this type of handshake.

The Dead Fish handshake says that the giver is unsure of himself or herself, unresponsive, nervous, and is not trustworthy. People will perceive you as a reserved and uninvolved type of a person if you give this type of handshake. The result is almost certain – the receiver will quickly want to get rid of your hand and anything that has to do with you. It will make potential business partners avoid you and push away social acquaintances from you.

The Glove

This is when you shake with one and cover the back of the receiver's hand with your other hand. Politicians are fond of using this type of handshake because it conveys a sense of authority or confidence. The Glove says that you are very self-confident. It can also mean that you are caring or sympathetic when used in a situation that requires condolence. If you not a politician, a minister, or if you are not trying to offer sympathy, please minimize the use of this type of handshake. In a business setting, this can portray you as being too desperate or overconfident unless you are in a position of authority (like an employer or a boss). Using this type of handshake for the opposite sex in a situation that does not require a show of sympathy or authority can make the other person think you are flirting with them.

Queen Fingertip

This is a type of handshake that involves offering the fingers to the other person as is commonly done between a queen and her subjects. This is common among many women, especially if they regard themselves as being higher in status than the other person.

The message of the Queen Fingertips is loud and clear: *"I am above you!"* or *"I don't regard or like you that much."* It can also portray you as someone who prefers their personal space because you are insecure. Use this handshake only when you truly want the other person to steer clear of you or if you are royalty.

The Pusher

When you shake someone's hand but extend your arms in such a way that it pushes the receiver away from you, or when you stretch your arms further away from your body during a handshake to create a significant gap between you and the receiver of the handshake, it is known as The Pusher.

This handshake has a similar attitude and message to the Queen's Fingertips. It says that you don't want others (or at least the receiver) getting into your personal space. If this is not the type of message you want to convey with your body language, please avoid The Pusher. However, if you want the other person to know that you respect their personal and emotional space or you want them to respect yours, you can use this handshake.

The Controller

A handshake that pulls the receiver's hand towards the giver is known as The Controller. It can also be a handshake where the receiver's hand is guided in a particular direction.

What this type of handshake conveys is that the giver is very controlling. If you do not want others to perceive you as domineering, then it is best to avoid this type of handshake. On the other hand, if you want the receiver to know that you are in charge, this is an excellent handshake to use. However, remember to keep a smile on your face while doing this so that you don't appear aggressive.

The Dominator

In this type of handshake, the giver places their hand on top of the receiver's palm instead of the usual handshake where both palms face sideways. This means the giver faces their palm down so that it covers the receiver's palm and remains on top of it for the duration of the handshake.

What The Dominator says is that you are superior and you dominate everything and everyone around you. If you want to portray a dominating image of yourself, this is the handshake to use. However, if you do not want to be perceived in that light, stick to the usual firm sideways-palm handshake.

The Submissive

The flip side of The Dominator is The Submissive handshake. The giver places their palm facing up while shaking the receiver.

This clearly says you are submissive to the other person. It can mean that you are loyal and humble, but it can also tell the other person that you are not confident of yourself, especially if it is used in a business or professional setting. An important client who is looking for a self-assured partner may likely not pick you if you give them this type of handshake.

Sweaty Palm

You may be very good at handshakes yet convey a negative message about yourself if you have sweaty palms. A sweaty palm screams nervousness and anxiety. It clearly tells the receiver that you are very uncomfortable or apprehensive. This can be a deal-breaker in a professional or business setting. In a social setting, it can put off a lot of potential acquaintances.

So, what do you do if you have palms that sweat naturally? Always keep a handkerchief or a paper towel close by and wipe your palms when you are meeting people. Of course, you should be discreet about this. Don't go wiping your palms in the presence of the person whom you want to shake hands with. That is body language that says you are clumsy!

Giving a Proper Handshake

Here are the steps you need to remember when giving a proper handshake. It may seem mechanical to follow these steps, but believe me, these steps will come naturally to you after some practice. And it doesn't matter if it is a professional or social setting, these steps work for all.

1. Extend your hand in front of you with your fingers straight and your palms facing sideways. Unless you are in a group that practice differently, the right hand is usually used for handshakes.

2. Firmly take hold of the other person's palm as if your palm is embracing theirs but without applying too much pressure.

3. Squeeze lightly while you gently shake their hand in an up and down movement twice or thrice.

4. Keep a smile on your face as you maintain eye contact with them. This shows that you are fully

present with them and you appreciate meeting them.

5. This last step is used when you are meeting someone for the first time. Introduce yourself with a confident tone of voice. For example, *"Hi, my name is..."* and then mention your name. You can add what you do but that is completely optional.

The whole of these steps takes anywhere between 3 to 6 seconds. Anything longer tends to signify flirting, aggression, or some other ulterior motive. The language of a proper handshake combined with eye contact and a great tone of voice can leave a good and lasting impression on the people you meet, especially for the first time.

Things to Avoid

When giving a handshake, avoid the following:

- Do not grab the receiver's hand in a clasping manner, yank it, and then release their hand in the name of a handshake. That is not an enjoyable experience for anyone.

- Don't vigorously shake people's hands throughout the duration of the handshake. Handshakes are meant to be mutual, so allow the other person to also have the chance to shake your hand.

- Don't ever pat your superior (employer, boss, or someone higher in authority) on the shoulder unless it is in private and the situation makes it proper for you to convey a feeling such as sympathy when they are in deep grief.

Practice Makes Perfect

Don't ignore the value of practicing. It may appear awkward, practicing a handshake with your close friends, but the time and effort you put into this will eventually pay off. So, practice giving a powerful handshake that will convey the right type of message you want.

Remember that it is possible to blunder your first few real-life attempts. This is okay. We learn from mistakes. Don't feel bad about it. Here's a quick tip you can use to cover up for your mistake: quickly give an honest compliment to the other person – say something nice about them, or simply ask a question to take their attention away from your seemingly poor handshake. Remember that they do not know what you are trying to achieve by the handshake; your motives are known only to you. So while your handshake may not have said you are a very self-confident person, the receiver may have only noticed that you are warm and welcoming (which isn't a bad message either).

Tips and Tricks about Handshakes

- **Initiating a Handshake**: No matter how self-confident you are, it is important to be sure about the rightness of initiating a handshake before you do so. In some settings or cultures, you are seen as rude if you initiate a handshake when meeting someone superior in status. In some other settings, it is seen as being proactive, bold, and self-assured. In order not to send the wrong signals to the people watching, ensure that you understand the setting in which you find yourself and then act appropriately. If you do not know how things work in a particular setting or culture, do not be shy to ask around.

- **Keep Your Hand Unoccupied**: You will be sending a message that says you are clumsy, socially unaware, or unapproachable if your hand is not readily available for a handshake. Trying to move stuff from one hand to the other or trying to find a good place to keep your stuff when the other person is already stretching their hand for a handshake is not a sign that you are ready to meet others. When it is obvious that you are going to meet others, make sure that you free one hand of all items that can hinder you from giving or receiving handshakes. Also, take your hands out of your pockets unless, of course, you do not want other people to approach you.

- **Unexpected Handshakes**: Sometimes someone can stretch their hand in a gesture of a handshake when you least expected it. Most of us are wired to immediately respond to an outstretched arm by also giving out our hands. This usually gives the other person the upper hand and makes them control the handshake (how long it lasts and in what direction it goes). Nevertheless, you can still take charge of such situations. When a handshake comes at you unexpectedly, switch to The Glove handshake – cover their hand with your other hand. This automatically slows down the giver's momentum and places you in control of the handshake.

- **Engage Your Elbows**: When you shake hands, make sure that you are engaging your elbow in your hand movement, not your wrist. If your hand movement is coming only from your wrist, your handshake will be flaccid and lacking in vitality.

- **Read the Other Person by their Hand**: Usually, the very first opportunity to make physical contact with a person you are just meeting happens during a handshake. This is an excellent opportunity to get a glimpse into the type of person they are. Do not let a handshake go by without trying to figure out what the other person may be like. Get a good feel of what their hand is telling you by making sure your own palms are not cupped but stretched out and your fingers are not curved. This way, you can read their personality to some extent in the brief moments which the handshake lasts.

- **Watch Your Posture**: It is important to be aware of your body posture when giving or receiving handshakes. When shaking hands in a seated position, make sure that your back is in an erect position so that you do not appear to be bowing to the other person unless they are royalty or the situation calls for it. Ensure that you have your feet planted firmly if you are in a standing position during a handshake. This will allow you to comfortably lean in slightly during the handshake, and lean out after the handshake. You can also break out of a handshake that is becoming uncomfortable for you by leaning out and stepping back a little bit so that the other person can break their hold.

- **Palm Facing Up**: When you are seated and trying to shake the hand of someone who is standing, you can face your palm up, especially if you are not sure that the other person will return the gesture. However, don't be too quick to use this gesture, as it can put you in a disadvantaged position.

- **Let Your Eyes Speak**: For a handshake to convey any meaningful message, the eyes have to be involved. During handshakes, make sure that you lock eyes with the other person briefly. This is a powerful way of complementing the message your hand is conveying. The energy of your hand combined with the passion, self-confidence, power, or respect in your eyes will deliver the most appropriate message.

Chapter 6: The Language of the Eyes

Recall that I mentioned in chapter 3 that I'll go into detail about the eyes in a subsequent chapter. Well, this right here is where we'll take a broader and deeper look into the various messages the eyes can convey. It isn't for lack of a proper description that the eyes are often referred to as the window to the soul. The eyes indeed have their own vocabulary that tends to convey messages for almost every emotional intention. This is why I have dedicated the whole of this chapter to explain in detail the language of the eyes.

It may not be possible to know the personality of someone by merely looking into their eyes, but they eyes let you have a glimpse into what they are thinking at that moment; and sometimes, that may be all the information you need to make an impact on the relationship you have with that person. The eyes are always saying something even when a person's face conveys a bland or blank expression. Notice that infants who have not even developed their ability for verbal communication can catch glimpses of subtle communication from the eyes of their parents and other adults.

By the end of this chapter, it is my hope that you would have learned how to assess a situation to determine the most appropriate eye movement to make in order to affect a positive outcome on the interactions you have with others.

Tips on Initiating Eye Contact

- **Respect other's need for privacy**. Staring at other people can feel like crowding their personal space. It is like beaming a spotlight on them when all they need is their privacy. You will unnerve and upset others if they are not open to making eye contact with you and you stubbornly continue to stare at them. In many cases, it makes you appear creepy, like a predator eyeing unwilling prey. Do not stare at people if they have made it abundantly clear that they don't want to make eye contact. They will know if you continue to stare even when they are not looking at you; they can sense your eyes on them.

- **Be discreet and sensitive about eye contact**. You don't have to lock eyes with the other person throughout your interaction in a bid to appear open, welcoming, or self-confident. Gauge their acceptance level and adjust your eye contact accordingly. Don't be too obvious about it. It is very okay to look away from them for a while.

- **Take the initiative.** Literally, initiate eye contact with the other person because people are most likely to avoid initiating eye contact. The general belief is that the other person may not like it. So, go ahead and initiate eye contact. The other person may look away initially, but give it another go and they will get the message that you are open to receiving eye contact. However, if they keep avoiding your eyes after three tries, allow them to. They may truly not want it or they may come around much later.

- **Never turn your eyes downward when you break your gaze**. Looking down when you break your gaze is an indication that you are submissive. In some other context, it could mean you are of low status or you feel shame. If you need to break your gaze, look to the left or right, but never down unless, of course, you intend to make the person feel superior.

- **Gently switch eyes**. When you glide your eye movement between the eyes of the other person, focusing on one eye for a bit and then gently traveling to the other eye in a smooth movement, the other person gets a sense that you are aware of them and paying close attention to them. But you have to be smooth about this. You don't want to be darting between the other person's eyes, as that can be very distracting and even confusing. And whatever you do, don't fix your gaze on the bridge of their nose. You will make the other person think that you are trying to manipulate them.

- **Practice with close people**. It is a good idea to first practice your eye movement with the people who are closest to you. Sometimes, we may not even be comfortable maintaining eye contact with family and friends. If you can't comfortably look into the eyes of someone you are used to, how do you expect to succeed with a stranger? So, go ahead and practice with a few family members and friends before moving on to other people.

Eye Movements and Possible Indications

Darting Eyes

Insecurity or discomfort can be detected by darting eyes. You cannot convey a message that says you are self-confident when your eyes keep darting to and fro. So, when you find yourself face to face with someone intimidating like your employer or someone you'll want to impress like the opposite sex, keep your eyes from moving back and forth.

Glancing Sideways

Glancing sideways can have two confusing emotional intentions. However, if you are diligent enough, you can spot the difference.

When someone looks sideways with a slightly raised eyebrow, it strongly suggests interest. It is possible that they even what to be intimate with you. But do not jump to conclusions without first taking the entire context into consideration.

Here's the other sideways look that can be easily confused with the one above. When someone glances sideways with a furrowed brow, it is an indication that they are not sure about something. It could also signify suspicion or they are being critical.

The slightly raised eyebrows and the furrowed brows are what differentiate these two sideways glances. Always remember this difference so that you do not confuse the two.

Raised Eyebrows

When someone raises their eyebrows while looking directly at you, it indicates a need for better communication. When you want the other person to clearly understand what you are saying, you can raise your eyebrows while looking directly at them. For example, try looking at your spouse when you are not talking about anything and then raise your eyebrows (not in a sexy way!). They are most likely to respond with a *"what?"* because they want to understand what you are communicating since there was no prior discussion or communication.

You can also use this to add extra emphasis to what you are saying. Here's something I'd like you to try in front of your bedroom mirror. Do not move your eyebrows as you look into the mirror and say the words, *"I hope you get my point?"* Now look into the mirror again and raise your eyebrows as you repeat the same words. You don't have to look too closely before you see clearly that the raised eyebrows throw in extra emphasis to your words.

Peering Eyes Over Glasses

Glasses give an impressive look to a woman, particularly in a business or professional setting. To make herself appear more impressive, she can peer at you from the top of her glasses. This is an excellent move for appearing intimidating, and it can be used both by women and men alike. Here's something that can add an extra effect to the intimidating move: use your index finger to pull down the glasses slightly.

Looking Down The Nose

Similar to the above eye movement, looking down your nose at someone is a way of telling them you are above them. You are telling the other person that you are fully in charge. If someone uses this move on you, they are showing their superiority over you.

Gazing

Depending on the context where gazing is used, it can convey strong disagreement, aggression, or intimacy. Gazing at the opposite sex may mean a deep interest in them. The same gaze, when directed at someone superior for a longer duration than usual, can mean aggression, opposition, or strong disagreement.

There are two invisible triangles on everyone's face where you can direct your gaze to provide the message you want to convey.

Imagine a line running from the left eye to the right eye and then converging at the forehead in a triangular shape. When you focus your gaze inside that triangle, you are telling the other person that you are in charge or you have authority over them. Staring inside that imaginary triangle is using the power gaze to stare them down.

The second imaginary triangle runs from the left eye to the right, forming the base of the triangle, and then converging at the mouth. When you stare into this triangle, you are clearly telling the other person that you care for them and support them. Fixing your gaze inside this triangle is using the social gaze to show comfort.

There is a third type of gaze that does not use an imaginary triangle. It is known as the intimate gaze. If you intend to send a clear message to the other person that you are having intimate thoughts about them, stare at their eyes and then gently move down to their mouth and gradually move your gaze to their body. When someone looks at you this way, they are sending you flirting signals.

Eye-blocking

Eye-blocking is a natural reaction to disgust. Observe a person who is blind from birth. Although they are blind, they will naturally cover their eyes when they hear some very repulsive or unpleasant news. This is an unconscious reaction.

So, when someone covers their eyes, it signifies being uncomfortable with something they have just heard or seen. Excessive blinking and excessive rubbing of the eyes are also types of eye-blocking.

Remembering Versus Lying Eyes

When someone is remembering something, their eyes move in a different direction than when they are lying. Looking up and then to the left is an indication that the person is trying to pry information from their memory. In other words, they are remembering something. On the flip side, looking up and then to the right is an indication that the person is engaging their imagination. In other words, they are not saying anything real; it's just lies.

Keep in mind that this doesn't work for everyone in the exact same way because we don't all have the same hand orientation; some people are right-handed while others are left-handed. For a left-handed person, their eye movements for remembering and lying are flipped.

Different Settings, Different Eye Contact

Showing Power

When you speak to someone on a one-on-one basis, make eye contact with them, but when it is their turn to speak, cut down the frequency of your eye contact. This is an excellent move to show that you have power or authority. When you make more eye contact while listening, it appears as if you are submissive. So, look at something else when someone whom you want to feel your power is talking to you and give them the occasional nod and grunt to let them know you are listening.

Power can also be shown through a stare down. Boxers and wrestlers use this eye contact a lot to stare down their opponent. If you intend to send a strong domineering message to someone, stare them down! Note, however, that you cannot improve the quality of your relationship with another person by staring them down. You can only make them submissive to you without necessarily being happy about it.

One other way to show power is to hide your eyes. Use mirror shades or dark shades to cover your eyes from passing along any message to the other person. The eye communication is only in one direction and it gives you the upper hand because you can see their eyes and read their intention but they cannot see yours. This power display can be observed with police officers who wear dark shades; they appear more intimidating than those who don't use dark shades.

Giving A Speech

Picture someone giving a speech in front of a small audience. They have their eyes glued to the paper in front of them and can hardly raise their head to look at the audience. Does that portray a self-confident person? Of course not!

When you make eye contact while giving a speech, you come across as someone who is sure of themselves. It makes you look trustworthy and competent. Your audience is likely to be open to receive your message when you make good eye contact with them.

Whether you are addressing a small or large audience, make actually eye contact with a few individuals in the audience. Do not ever heed the advice which suggests that you should look above the head of the people in your audience. They will know that you are avoiding their gaze and that can discredit the message you are trying to pass.

When you look at your audience, try not to pan or sweep over them from one end to the other and then return the eye movement again. Be natural. Look at one individual as you talk, and then gradually switch to other people in the audience just as you would do if you were talking to them one-on-one. Also, remember to either memorize your speech or make note of the important points so that you do not have to keep darting your eyes back and forth from the audience to your notes.

During Interviews

If you are attending an interview, you will need to strike a balance between making eye contact and looking away. Too much eye contact can blow your chances of being picked and too little eye contact can equally ruin your chances. No company will want to employ someone who lacks confidence – which is what your body language will convey if you avoid eye contact with the interviewer.

Professional or Business Setting

You cannot effectively sell anything – a product or an idea – if you avoid eye contact with your client. No one is going to close a deal with a sales rep that has shifty eyes. So, make sure that your eyes are on your clients when you are brokering a deal with them. If they should raise any questions, meet their eyes while you answer their questions. This is a clear signal to them that you are trustworthy.

If you are making a presentation before a board of executives, for example, don't focus only on the authority figure. Make sure you bring everyone along so that they all get a sense of being part of the meeting.

Chapter 7: Rapport Building Techniques

Understanding body language goes beyond the ability to properly read the subtle non-verbal cues that abound in daily human interactions. Reading body language is just one part of the equation. The other half of this knowledge has to do with how to deliberately and properly encode messages into body language. The key words to note are deliberately and properly.

In this chapter, we shall take a look at how to say a ton of persuasive things without using words. This will help you get along well with other people even if they are just meeting you for the very first time. In order to get along well with others, you do not need to pretend to be something you are not; neither do you need to please them with your body language. However, you can use pretense in a positive way. In a later chapter, we shall learn how to effectively fake your body language to influence others positively. But for now, let us see how to use non-verbal cues to build a strong rapport with others even if they are total strangers. We shall focus on using the most effective body language technique – the chameleon effect, or body mirroring – for this purpose.

Using The Chameleon Effect to Quickly Build Rapport

Firstly, you need to understand that rapport is the ability to affect someone else in a positive way so that they have a strong feeling that you understand and connect with them on a deep level. You can build a strong rapport with other people if you learn how to stealthily use the chameleon effect on others. The chameleon effect means mirroring two major aspects of a person's non-verbal cues: their body posture/gestures and their tone of voice.

If you can perfect your ability to mirror these two aspects of a person's body language, then you can blend in with just about anyone you fancy. Here's how to properly use these tools.

Connect

First, establish a connection with the other person. As you interact with others, learn to gauge your connection level with them. If you don't feel any connection to them, there is a good chance that they too don't feel any connection with you. Here's how to establish a connection with the other person: Give your undivided attention to them for the duration of your interaction. Take your attention away from distractions such as your mobile phone, laptop, TV, or whatever it is that can cause distractions. Make eye contact with the person from time to time. If it is not possible to stand or sit directly in front of them, ensure that you are at least in their line of view. Additionally, give them encouraging nods to show your attentiveness. Doing all of this is bound to establish a connection between you and them. Once you have done this, proceed to the next step.

Copy the Speech Pattern

The next thing to do after establishing a connection with the other person is to mimic their speech pattern. Now I do not mean to start talking exactly like the other person. Mimicking speech pattern means to observe the pace with which they talk, whether it is fast or slow, note whether their voice is calm or loud, and then adjust your voice tone to suit theirs. If you share the same accent as the other person, that is a plus for you. Copying the pace and tone of voice of the other person can easily go unnoticed by the other person, more so than copying their body movements. Nevertheless, speech pattern mimicry has the same influencing effect as copying body movements. If you can copy both the speech pattern and the body movements without being apparent, that would be ideal.

Observe the Punctuator

We all have a punctuator we use during conversations. This is a simple body movement we have grown accustomed to and use frequently, especially when we are trying to buttress our conversational points. For some, it could be raising the eyebrows, and for others, it could be some form of hand gesture. Whatever it is, you will discover it if you pay close attention to the other person as they speak and interact.

Once you find what their punctuator is, use it when you are showing your agreement with something they have said or implied. Here's an example: a person who punches their fist into the open palm of their other hand as their punctuator will bond with you easily when you show your agreement using the same punctuator. Agreeing with them while saying something like, *"That's absolutely right!"* as you punch your fist into your open palm sends a subtle message to their mind that you are like them in many ways.

So, look out for finger snaps, finger pointing, a clap, or any other frequently used punctuator and mimic that cautiously. You do not need to study a person for a long time to know their punctuator. This is why you can use this to make an instant connection with a total stranger.

Put it to Test

This last step is optional. You can test to see if you have really established a bond with the other person. Keep in mind that the test should be done only once or twice, or else it may become obvious to the other person that you have been watching their body movements.

To test the bond or connection, do something with your body that is not related to the conversation you are having with them. If they mirror your body movement, you have successfully established a bond. Cash in on that and strengthen the connection. Here's an example of several body movements you can use to test your connection.

- Slightly tilt your head.

- Scratch an imaginary itch on the side of your face.

- Play with your ear lobe for a few seconds.

- If you are sitting down, cross or uncross your legs.

- Interlace your fingers.

Rapport Building Tips to Remember

Be Ready to Impact Others Positively

Being yourself is a great idea, but if being yourself is wearing a long face, looking shabby, and carrying an air of doom and gloom, then you're not going to get very far in your attempt to build a strong rapport with others. The people you meet with, whether for the first time or not, will judge you from what they see and perceive about your personality. It doesn't matter if you are a good person on the inside; if your outward expression doesn't match the goodness inside of you, there is no way the people around you can see that inward goodness.

I'd strongly suggest that you create a very positive impression of yourself on others, especially if you are meeting them for the first time. Although not everyone is given to being judgmental or critical about others, there is an unconscious part of all of us that wants to form an opinion about the personality of the people we are meeting. Therefore, give people a good impression of yourself by your mood and physical appearance. If they sense energy, vigor, and liveliness in you, they are likely to be drawn to you and build a strong rapport with you over time. On the other hand, if they sense an unfriendly demeanor about you, they will repel you.

The different people you meet on a daily basis are the connection you need for the next level in your career, personal relationships, and every other aspect of your life. This is because you need other humans to live a happy life. If you blow your chance to connect with these people, you may end up living an unhappy life for a long time.

Don't Ignore the Basics

What would be the use of showing up beaming with a confident smile and then having a handshake that lacks matching energy? What good is an immaculate dress when you cannot look at the other person in the eye? What would be the point of going through the rigors of looking good and confident, and then not paying attention to the person you are meeting?

I'm sure you get the point I'm making. The very basics of body language reading which we have discussed in the previous chapters are all essential to building rapport. They all work together to give you the type of persona you'll be proud of. So, do your best to remember and apply them in your interactions with the people around you.

Here's something you should also remember: don't try so hard to impress others. When you are meeting with others, don't go overboard in trying to build rapport with them such that you are all over the place at the same time. You don't have to talk continuously about every single topic. It is not necessary to show that you know a thing just because you want to appear likeable. Non-stop conversations will make you appear too desperate. Be moderate in your interactions. Allow some room for brief silence during your interaction with others. Give them some room to also communicate verbally and non-verbally. That way, you get an opportunity to read and discover their emotional intentions.

Remember that you are not just out looking for people to read; you should also be mindful of what your non-verbal cues are saying to others around you. The last thing you want is to lose yourself in the search to understand others. So, while you are trying to figure out if the other person is self-confident, make sure you are not appearing arrogant. And while trying to determine if the next person is calm and collected, ensure that you are not coming across as tensed and anxious.

Focus on the Things You Share in Common

You cannot successfully build rapport with others if you keep on bringing up the things that differentiate you from them. Your focus should be on highlighting the things that you share in common with the other person. For example, if you are meeting someone for the first time and you discover that they are passionate about ballet dancing just as you are, cash in on that and share your passion for ballet dancing with them. It will seem as if you've known each other forever! Although you may not like every single thing the other person likes, the more time you spend finding out what things both of you like in common, the better the quality of your relationship with them will be.

Show Empathy

People tend to lean towards those who understand them on some deeper level. You cannot build rapport with another person if you don't have some form of empathy with them. If you can leverage the knowledge that humans have an innate need to be understood, you will be amazed at the number of strong connections you have built with others in a relatively short period of time.

Your ability to see the world from another person's perspective will open you up to more opportunities than you can imagine. That ability will make you an empathetic person who can easily understand and connect with others as if you have known them all their lives.

I am not implying that you let go of your own personal views and perspectives because you want to appear welcoming and accommodating to others. Remember, you do not have to lose yourself in the quest to understand others! What I am advocating is for you to put yourself in other people's shoes in order to see things from their perspective. This is an essential part of building rapport.

When you can connect easily with others, you open yourself to the resources hidden inside the people around you. You are not doing anything unethical by building a strong rapport with others so as to benefit from it, because it is a win-win situation that is mutually beneficial. What you are doing is building a rich social network that serves everyone involved.

Chapter 8: Attraction Body Language

When there is chemistry (not the one taught in schools) between two people, they like each other and that can result in an intimate relationship. In this chapter, we shall take a look at the things that women and men do that strengthen the attraction bond (or chemistry) between both sexes. If you are already in a relationship, this chapter will help to improve the quality of your relationship using attraction body language. And if you are hoping to attract someone into your life, this might be just the tool you need. Let us begin with the ladies before we move on to the gentlemen, shall we?

How to Make a Man Like You

Ladies, the tips and tricks here may not all work in the same way for every single man; remember that all men are not the same. *"Men are all the same!"* is a conclusion rooted deeply in blind generalization by brokenhearted women. Therefore, I strongly suggest that you take a little time to understand the type of man in your life or the type of man you are hoping to attract. However, on a general note, there are some things that tend to catch the interest of most men, and here they are:

1. **Putting on his shirt**. Slide into his shirt and wear it over your bare legs. Let most of the shirt buttons be left undone. Don't dress in his clothes as if you are going for some serious outing. Be as casual as you can be in his clothes. Men trip for these things!

2. **Being nice to random people, especially the elderly and kids**. When a man sees a woman's maternal instinct in action, like when she treats a random kid nicely, he is drawn to

her. The same thing goes for treating elderly people with kindness and respect. Men are generally attracted to women who are kind hearted.

3. **Shaving his face**. The act of shaving a man's face speaks more intimately than any words you can ever tell him. You don't have to be a great barber or even get it right. As a matter of fact, you do not have to complete the shaving. Just begin and even play around with the shaving cream. Rub some on his nose and have a good laugh together. You may even feign a serious face for a while to appear as if you are giving him an excellent shave, meanwhile, you are simply giving him an uneven shave. And if you happen to be good at it, he may never visit a barber's shop ever again!

4. **Biting the lip**. Okay, this one is very sexy to most men. When a woman bites her lip, it gives her a helpless look that activates the man's inborn desire to protect her. It also makes her look very sexy. So, whether you are biting your

lip or the man's lip, men will fall for this move.

5. **Having deep conversations**. This may not seem sexy, but men look out for a woman who can participate in their intellectual development. While looking sexy can attract a man, if the quality of your conversation is shallow or leans only towards romance, the man may tire out quickly. A man is very attracted to a woman who can inspire him and nudge him towards achieving his life's goals through deep and meaningful conversation.

6. **Whispers and winks**. A playful woman is a man's delight! Winking at a man unexpectedly or whispering in his ear, especially in public places, are some of the playful things that most men find very attractive in women. When you make playful faces or goof around the house once in a while, you make your man want to spend more time with you. When he recalls your playful face, it brings a warm smile to his face and heart, too!

7. **Being friends with his friends**. Men are always torn between their better halves and their friends. If a woman makes it easier for the man by befriending the man's friends, she mends that tear and the man adores her more. So, look for common ground between you and your man's friends and explore that to become a prominent part of his life both at home and when he's out with his friends, which you happen to be also.

8. **Telling the story behind a scar or tattoo**. Women go through a great deal to make sure that their skin remains flawless. This is why it catches a man's attention if a woman turns her skin into a canvass. When a man shows interest in your tattoo or looks at a scar on your skin, go into a brief story of why you choose to get your skin tattooed or how you got the scar. You are using this opportunity to tell the man about yourself. So, make it an interesting story— without exaggerating, of course.

9. **Working out**. Women tend to be drawn to

men with great abs and good body muscles. The same thing applies to men. When most men see a woman working out, it turns on their interest level. Perhaps it has to do with the woman's curvatures being accentuated during workouts. Or maybe it has to do with the sense of being mindful of her body weight and physiology. Whatever it is, men tend to be attracted to a woman who works out.

10.   **Laughing at his jokes even when they are not funny**. When a woman laughs, men like it. They see that they are able to affect a positive response from you. So, laugh at a man's humor and you are steadily working your way into his heart. Even when a woman patronizes a man by laughing at his dry jokes, the man is most likely to ignore the patronizing attitude because her laughter boosts his manliness.

How to Make a Woman Like You

To the men, there is no one universal body language to make a woman like you because, like men, women too are wired differently. While verbalizing your feelings can make a woman like you, what you do can have a farther-reaching effect than the words you speak. Women are generally known to fall for the following male actions.

1. **Doing chores**. First on this list is something that is not necessarily romantic but has the capacity to make a woman fall head over heels for you. Home chores are usually considered to be a woman's role. So when you, as a man, perform chores like doing the dishes at home, collecting her laundry (or the family's laundry), mopping the floor, bathing the kids, and any other home chore, these little things can make a woman really like you.

2. **Fixing things**. You don't have to be an expert or a professional to fix little things around the house. Many women consider being handy as

sexy for reasons men cannot really fathom. So, roll up your sleeves, get your hands dirty, and fix those broken little things around the house. She'll appreciate you more!

3. **Rolling your sleeves to the elbow**. Talking about rolling up your sleeve to fix things, many women find the act of rolling up your shirt sleeve to the elbow sexy. Why this is so may not be easily understood by men, but it works. So, even if you are not trying to get things around the house fixed, wait to be with her and then take your time to gradually roll up your shirt sleeves to your elbow. Be deliberate about this act, and you may end up turning her on! One more thing: this works better with buttoned-up shirts than with other types of men's clothing like sweaters.

4. **Make her laugh**. If you can make a woman laugh genuinely, she will be attracted to you. If she's already in a relationship with you, she'll like you more. You don't have to be a comedian to make her laugh. Just be confident about your

style of humor and you're good to go. Make sure not to overdo this because you can easily tire her out. Look for appropriate times to chip in with a little humor.

5. **Listening to her**. Pay attention to a woman when she speaks, even if it is a passing conversation. If you remember the seemingly little details she has shared with you, she'll get a sense of being an important part of your life. Generally, it is believed that women talk more than men and men listen less than women do. If you can break out of this generally held belief and listen intently to her when she speaks, it will be a huge plus for you.

6. **Spending quality time with kids**. When a woman sees you having fun with kids or chatting and explaining things to them, it triggers an evolutionary signal in her that you can make a great dad; and women love great dads!

7. **Doing random romantic acts**. Men usually

think that being romantic is expensive, so they spend all the time they have working hard to save enough money to take the woman they like on a trip or to the most expensive restaurant in town. The problem with this is that it takes an awfully long time before many men can afford this type of romantic act. Women actually value the little acts that show that you care. For example, bringing her a cup of coffee while she's still in bed, helping the kids with their homework so that she can concentrate on her work, helping her dry her hair without her asking, and lots of other little things can be very romantic without being expensive.

8. **Reacting softly to other women and animals**. Women take note of how you react to and treat other women. If you are rude to your mom or a waitress, for example, the woman in your life will take note. If you are a softy for animals, for example, a kitten, she'll also notice. She'll form an opinion about who you are based on how you treat other women and how kind

you are to animals.

9. **Be passionate about something**. It doesn't matter what your passion is, just find it and put your energy into it. A woman wants a man that is passionate about something – just about anything! So, put your energy into that hobby or dream and work at developing it if you want to keep your woman interested in you.

10. **Offer her your coat**. Offering your coat to a woman on a cold night in a condescending way will not make her like you. On the other hand, kissing her hand and bowing like a prince in shining armor while offering her your coat won't do the trick either. A woman wants to be treated nicely but in a courteous manner. So, offer her your coat in a polite way and if it is appropriate, gently brush strands of hair out of her face before she steps out into the cold.

Chapter 9: Reading Advanced Body Language

Some non-verbal cues are subtler and more elusive to read than others. Earlier in chapter 3, I introduced you to some of the basic body movements and what they could possibly indicate, but body movements can be more complex than that. For this reason, I have written this chapter to explain the more evasive non-verbal cues that can easily go unnoticed. Getting a good knowledge of these subtler body movements will help you reach better conclusions about the emotional intent of others.

As always, context and cluster are very important when drawing conclusions from non-verbal cues. You do not want to base your judgment on "circumstantial evidence," rather, what you want is to take into consideration the particular situation that surrounds the expression of the non-verbal cue and also take note of other cues so that you can arrive at a more informed conclusion.

There is no hard and fast rule about this; remember, it is not an exact science. Human beings are very complex and can go to great lengths to mask their true intentions. As a matter of fact, someone who knows about body language can successfully hide their true intentions since they know what you are looking out for. For example, knowing the language of the eyes (as we have seen in chapter 6), you can successfully initiate and maintain eye contact with another person even when you are lying. You know that people who lie tend to have shifty eyes or try to avoid eye contact, so you can deliberately falsify your eye movement to depict a different thing from what you are actually doing.

All these notwithstanding, I have listed some of the subtler non-verbal cues below together with the intention they are likely to point to.

Increased Legs and Feet Movement

I have earlier mentioned that intentions can be easily masked away from other body parts, but are a bit more difficult to hide away from the feet. Beyond the sign of interest or disinterest that can be revealed from the direction where someone's feet are pointing, there are other subtle messages that can be picked up by simply observing someone's feet.

A person's legs and feet can convey anxiety, stress, and uneasiness by the way they move them around. For example, when you are having a talk with your child and they begin to wind their feet around the chair where they are seated or around any piece of available furniture, that is a high indication that they are not at ease. In cases where there is no furniture close by, a person under stress is likely to wind their legs around each other or make shuffling movements with their feet. If you notice this type of leg and feet movement when you are questioning someone (a junior colleague, your child, your student, etc.), the other person is probably not letting you in on the complete information. There's more to the story they are feeding you at that moment.

Here's a way to observe someone's legs and feet movement, especially during questioning: let them take their seat where you can have a direct view of their whole body. If there's a table between you, remove it or sit away from the table so that you can clearly see their legs and feet.

Sitting Face-to-Face

Assuming a face-to-face sitting position conveys attentiveness. This work both ways: you can use this sitting position to let the other person get a message that says you are keenly aware of them and paying attention to them, and you can also read the same message from someone who sits facing you directly.

However, in some situations, it may not be possible to sit directly facing the other person. In such situations, you can turn your body towards the other person. And if you are the person doing the talking and you notice someone turning their body towards you even when their sitting position makes it not possible to sit facing you directly, their body language is a clear indication that they are paying close attention to you.

Nevertheless, do not confuse paying attention with agreement. Someone may be paying rapt attention to you because they are looking for slips and contradictions in what you are saying. The body language for agreement is quite different from the body language of attentiveness.

Uncrossing Arms and Legs

There is something about the crossing of the arms and legs that indicates a blockage. It is an unconscious way the body blocks or defends itself against anything (ideas, information, or physical attack) it perceives as threatening or unwelcome.

Here's something you should try out the next time you are talking with someone or a group of people (such as during a presentation): Observe if the other person or the audience you are speaking to have their arms and legs crossed. If they do, pause your talk or presentation and ask them to uncross their limbs or do something to make them uncross their arms and legs.

Uncrossed arms and legs have been found to improve memory. As you are well aware by now, arm crossing is a defensive body language, so a large chunk of what you say to someone who has their arms and legs crossed will hardly remain in their memory after the interaction.

Stealing a Quick Glance at the Time

If you are engrossed in whatever it is you are saying, you may hardly notice when someone makes this body movement. A quick glance at the time strongly suggests that the other person needs to be somewhere equally important or has another appointment they need to keep.

If you happen to be making a presentation to a group of people, it is very important to note the body movements of the people you are talking to in addition to focusing on making a great presentation. If your attention is not on their body movements, you will miss out on a whole lot of information they are silently passing to you.

When you observe this quick glance at the clock or wristwatch, whether it is in a one-on-one conversation or talking to a group of people, take the cue and wrap up your talk. Prolonging your topic is merely wasting both yours and their time.

On the flip side, you can use this movement to encode a *"summarize your points"* message to another person. Nevertheless, do not use this for someone who is above or superior to you in an official or professional setting. That will be considered as insubordination or rudeness to your superior.

Smiling

A smile on the face can easily be construed as a sign of friendliness. However, this is not always the case. A person who wears a smile too frequently may be signifying that they are submissive. For example, a subordinate in a work environment may want to remain in the good books of his boss and therefore flashes a smile ever so frequently that it unconsciously says, *"I am loyal to you."* As a boss, if you are on the lookout for people who will go the extra mile for you, these are the people you should enlist.

On the other hand, smiling too frequently can give you away as being weak and feeble minded. If you do not want to come across as such, you will do well to consciously play down your smiles. For example, a woman may consider a man to be courteous if he wears a smile once in a while during their interaction. But if he continues to have a smile pasted on his face, she may begin to think of him as a weakling and a loser!

Here's something else about a smile that can easily pass unnoticed. When someone has a smile on their face that does not reveal their teeth, it is known as a tight-lipped smile. It may pass as a genuine smile, but it really is not. It usually indicates that the person wearing that smile is not giving their candid opinion. For example, someone may say something nice about your new hairstyle and follow it with a tight-lipped smile. It is very likely that they did not give you their honest opinion about that hairstyle. While it may not automatically mean that they don't like you or are not happy for you, they may simply not want to hurt your feelings by telling you their honest opinion. The tight-lipped smile can also indicate that the person wearing it doesn't like your company but they do not want to appear rude by telling you off.

And while we are still on the subject of a smile, it can also be used to indicate sarcasm. This is what the facial expression of a smirk signifies. It is usually a smile mixed with a frown, but because the teeth are showing, it appears like a smile. When you observe this on the face of the person you are talking with, something you have said doesn't ring true with them but they are trying to make you think they agree with you.

The Battle Stance and Chin Jut

Anger and aggression do not only show up on the face. When someone stands with their feet apart, firmly planted on the floor, and their hands on their hips, do not rush into the conclusion that they are assuming the power pose (check out chapter 1o for the power pose). Remember that for an accurate body language reading, you need to look out for clusters. Look at their chin: are they pushing it out? If they are they, it is definitely not a power pose; instead, it is the battle stance and it is an indication of anger and rage (moreover, the power pose is usually something a person does in private).

In personal relationships, it is very common to find women using the battle stance to indicate rage against their spouse or children. Men do not use the battle stance very often, although the chin jut is common among both sexes.

In a professional setting, both the battle stance and the chin jut are not very common. People are expected to behave very maturely at work, so they will usually act civil even when they are boiling inside! However, during intense pressure, the façade may come off and this body language may be displayed. And because adults are expected to be civil, they may not resort to physical assault (unless in an abusive relationship) but they can give in to using hurtful words to calm their rage.

If you ever notice this body language, do all you can to quickly interject a different topic or quietly find a way to end the discussion immediately. It is a good idea to allow some time to pass in order to make the other person calm down. But in cases where it becomes necessary to continue the discussion, channel the talk towards finding a truce or pacifying the other person or those involved.

Chapter 10: Faking Your Body Language

Many people have misconceptions about faking body language. It seems the intent for faking body language is always for negative or unethical purposes, but that is not always the case and certainly isn't the reason I have included it in this chapter. To be clear, we all fake our body language at one time or the other during the course of our interactions with others. We do this most times unconsciously, and it is aimed at manipulating others. The purpose of this chapter is to teach you how to convert this unconscious manipulation into something you can do at will.

Another misconception is on the idea of manipulation. When you hear the word manipulate, it is very likely that you have all your defenses up and scream foul play! Nevertheless, I'd like you to view manipulation from a different angle. Here are two quick examples that will help you shift your perspective about manipulation.

Mrs. X wants her daughter to have lots of fun on her prom night. Her daughter's dress did not fit quite well but as soon as she emerged from her room, Mrs. X beamed at her with a warm smile and an expression on her face that says, *"You are perfect!"* Her daughter feels really great about her dress and had lots of fun at her prom party without noticing whatever was wrong with her dress.

Miss Y wants Sally to look bad in front of her classmates. She made jeering faces at Sally and looked spitefully at her shoes. Sally's classmates began looking at her shoes and Sally began feeling self-conscious as she walked to her seat. She was in a bad mood for the rest of the day.

In the first example, Mrs. X manipulated her daughter to make her feel great even when the conditions were not so great. In the second example, Miss Y manipulated Sally to feel bad. In both examples, manipulation was used as a tool to influence another person's feelings and behavior, but one had a positive outcome and the other had a negative one. The real issue is not with the tool (manipulation) used; rather, the issue is with the intention with which the tool was used.

For the purpose of this book, I want you to view faking body language as a manipulative tool which is aimed at deliberately influencing another person into a mutually beneficial behavior for all involved. I am not in any way encouraging anyone to fake their body language as a means to defraud, hurt, or cause harm to another person.

How to Fake Body Language Effectively

I'm sure you have heard the phrase *"Fake it till you make it!"* It is usually intended to boost a belief in oneself even when things are not going as planned. This is a powerful phrase that is very true also for your body language. There is a connection between your physical body posture and the chemicals in your brain. Assuming certain postures will make your brain release chemicals (hormones) into your body and make you feel vulnerable, anxious, or even downright fearful. There are other postures too that will automatically trigger a release of self-confidence building hormones into your body and you will almost immediately begin to feel really confident in yourself.

In order to become really good at faking your body language to the point where you can easily fool almost anyone, I'd recommend that you apply the following tips. They appear simple, but their impact over time is amazingly powerful. Keep in mind that if you are not convinced about your own performance, it will be difficult to convince others with your performance.

1. Create short videos of yourself in different situations as you interact with others. Several 5 to 10-minute videos will do just fine. During the recording, completely ignore the fact that you are making a video and be as natural as you can. When you watch the videos, turn off the volume so that you can only see your gestures, movements, and expressions. Notice the message your body is passing across and try to determine if that is exactly what you intended to say in those situations. Can you improve the way your body conveys the message? Is there a way you can successfully conceal some of the

messages your body (face, hands, head movements, and so on) is conveying? Studying your body language this way will help you improve it to either convey more or less information. This is a crucial step in the art of faking your body language.

2. Another way to effectively fake your body language which deals more with boosting self-confidence is by learning the art of being present. Whether it is a professional or social meeting, right before you make contact with someone you are expecting or get into a meeting, take deep breaths for some minutes and bring your attention to your immediate environment. Let go of the thoughts of the meeting or its outcome and simply focus on the present moment. You can clench and unclench your fists to stop any shakiness. This practice will make you calmer and remove any anxiety that may exist in you. It is in this calmer mood that you can become really aware of what your body movements

are saying during the meeting or contact with the other person.

Okay, let's now turn our attention to some real-life situations that will require you to use your body language to influence others. If you practice the steps above, you will not find it difficult to call up any non-verbal cues you want to put on display at a moment's notice. In short, if you practice well, you will be able to appear very confident even if you are very nervous inwardly, show proper interest in anyone even if you are not the least interested in them, and make others feel relaxed or comfortable when they are around you.

How to Properly Fake Interest in Others

Every now and then, people get the classic advice to show interest in others even when they apparently aren't interested.

Question: How do you show interest when you are not interested in any way?

Answer: By faking the body language of interest!

But before you start to stare or gaze and someone and vigorously nodding to show interest, you need to first understand the human attention span because it is directly linked to the capacity to show interest in anything. Normal human beings do not keep their attention on one particular subject for long periods at a stretch. At some point, our attention is likely to be distracted by something else or we will just get bored and lose interest. With this in mind, here's how to fake interest in others:

1. Don't overdo it! Appear obviously interested but don't keep your attention on the other person 100% of the time. Here's a rule of thumb to guide you; maintain eye contact with the other person for a few seconds and look away. Look at their face (not eyes) for a few minutes and look away.

2. Nod calmly and use words like, "*I'm with you*" or "*keep going*" while you quickly look at something else or quickly do something else. Make sure you keep interjecting your

focus on them with something very brief and please do this cautiously. Too many interjections will also mean that you are not paying attention to them and therefore, not interested in them or what they are saying. You need to find a balance between showing too much interest and faking distraction once in a while during the interaction. If you are having a short interaction, it is better not to have more than one or two fake distractions.

3. Here's something that will make anyone believe that you are completely interested in them even if you aren't paying attention to them the whole time. If the other person was interrupted or distracted during your conversation or discussion, make a habit of trying to continue the conversation from where they stopped even if you weren't listening at all. Here's how: when the distraction is over, say something like, "*So, you were trying to say something about ...*"

and allow them to complete your sentence and continue from there.

4. Don't ask for a favor immediately after you give someone a compliment. It tells them your compliment was insincere and a means to lure them into doing you the favor. No one likes being taken for a fool, so don't ever do that. If you really want to ask for a favor but need to warm up to the person first, do so after you have engaged in quite a bit of conversation, especially if you are not too familiar with the person. Keep an open body posture – hands out of your pocket, showing your palms as you speak, not crossing your arms on your chest, slightly raising your eyebrows to show interest, and so on – during your interaction and gently guide the conversation towards the favor you need to ask.

How to Make Others Feel Comfortable Around You

One huge advantage of faking body language is that you can easily build a strong bond between you and others. The truth is that as you continue to practice body language to influence others into liking you or at least being comfortable with you, you will eventually become so good at it that your body language will no longer be fake. It will become second nature. When this happens, you have successfully faked it until you made it! Here are some tips and tricks to make people feel at ease with you.

Smile

Smiling is a universal language that everyone, including infants, understands. It has the capacity to make others feel welcomed. So, you can use a smile (real or fake) to disarm someone, influence them into letting down their guard, and make them feel at ease around you.

However, even though a smile is perhaps the simplest of all non-verbal cues to read, faking a smile is not as simple as it looks. A genuine smile occurs as a result of impulses from your brain. These impulses signal specific groups of muscles located on your lips and eyes among other places on your face. This is what is responsible for micro-expressions which are very difficult to fake because you cannot fake the impulses controlling micro-expression.

To properly use a fake smile to influence another person positively, I will suggest the following:

- Smile from a good distance away from the other person. This will make it difficult for them to detect if it is a fake smile, since you are not close enough for them to clearly read your face.

- If you are in a situation where you cannot put a reasonable enough distance between you and the other person (like when you are seated face to face with them), simply let the smile flash quickly across your face. Don't let it remain pasted on your face for more than a couple of seconds, or else it will give you away!

- You don't have to show your teeth when you are wearing a fake smile. Your face will look very clumsy if you show your teeth during a fake smile. Simply raise your eyebrows slightly for more effect instead of showing your teeth.

Effective Listening

Remember what I said about the human attention span? If you can keep that in mind, you should be able to successfully fake the body language that makes you appear as if you are effectively listening to other people. The problem with trying to fake effective listening is that the average person tends to overdo it. There is nothing wrong with appearing as if you are paying rapt attention. The problem, however, is that when you do that from the beginning of your interaction to the end without as much as taking a slight break from the act, you are going to spook the other person (*his interest if far beyond what I'm saying! What is he up to?*). Or, they will easily catch on to what you are doing.

So, here are the non-verbal cues you should work on to convey to the other person you are really into whatever it is they are saying.

- Nod occasionally to tell the other person that you are getting their point of view. A nod is also a silent language that tells the other to keep on talking.

- Nodding too much is a dead giveaway that you are merely pretending to listen. It can also mean that you are trying to seek favor from the other person (usually someone in a higher position of power like your boss). Excessive nodding can be interpreted as flattery and instead of making the other person comfortable around you, it can push them far away from you.

- Squint your eyes as you nod slowly to paint a picture that you are deeply thinking about what the other person is saying.

- To add an extra effect, rub your index finger along the side of your face, or rub your thumb under your chin all the while making low "*hmm*" sound. This is a very powerful non-verbal cue that indicates deep thought. Combining this move with the eye squint and a slow nod is the perfect killer move for making anyone relax and share their deepest thoughts with you!

The Chameleon Effect (Body Mirroring)

We tend to like those who are like us. If you can be like the chameleon – faking every environment you find yourself in at will – then you would have stumbled on the key to make people like you or feel comfortable around you.

The chameleon effect, as I've earlier explained in chapter 7, is another term for mirroring another person's non-verbal cues. However, instead of focusing only on their body gestures, mirroring goes a step further to copy the other person's tone of voice, too. Mimicking another person's gestures, tone of voice, body angle, posture, and facial expressions is a great way to subliminally send messages to their unconscious mind to make them see that you have several things in common and will eventually make them more relaxed and comfortable around you.

If there is one technique that can easily give you away, it is this one. If every time your friend, colleague, boss, partner, or whoever it is you are interacting with changes their body posture you immediately copy their move, they will know that you are mimicking their moves and think you are creepy. Remember, coping moves like a robot will defeat the goal you are trying to achieve. Here's what to keep in mind when using the chameleon effect or mirroring.

- Don't copy every single move the other person makes.

- Time your moves to be a couple of minutes behind theirs.

- Let your body movements flow naturally and let them correlate with what you are saying.

- If you are meeting a person for the first time, mimic their tone of voice. However, if it is someone whom you've known for a long time, like your friend, partner, or work colleague, it may not be wise to copy their tone of voice.

They already know how you speak, so faking it won't work with them. Nevertheless, you can copy some of their punctuators. If you don't know what a punctuator is, kindly go back to chapter 7 and read the tips I shared about building a strong rapport.

Use Their Name

A person's name is something very personal. When you use it (tactfully), you are connecting with the person on a deeper level and making them more open to trusting you. When you mention a person's name while talking to them, you personalize what you are saying to them. For example, saying *"Here's a glass of water, Sally"* has more effect than saying *"Here's a glass of water."*

Whether or not the person is a stranger does not stop you from using this technique. In fact, if you can use a complete stranger's name during your conversations, it is a huge plus for you. You make them feel that you paid attention right from the beginning when they introduced themselves.

How to Fake Self-Confidence

One of the more common uses for faking body language is to convey a sense of self-confidence (even if you are lacking it). Right from childhood, parents encourage their kids to fake the body language of self-confidence, especially when the kids have to deal with bullies. The good thing about this practice is that its effects are not only meant to manipulate other people, but it actually increases your confidence level in real-life.

In order to effectively fake self-confidence body language, you'll need to learn to use the following.

Claiming Your Territory

Timid or fearful people seem to cramp themselves into a corner. On the other hand, confident people tend to occupy a lot of space. This is what you should have in mind when faking the body language of self-confidence. So, when you stand or sit, claim your space – spread yourself to occupy your territory!

In a standing position, let your hands be on your hips or loosely hanging by your side with your head held high. If you are standing in front of a desk or table, lean in and place your palm facing down on the table top as you hold the gaze of the other person.

In a sitting position, make sure your feet are apart and planted firmly on the floor. Let your arms come to rest on the armrest or spread them on a table in front of you. Alternatively, place one hand over the top of your chair. All of these are excellent ways to hide any fear or anxiety that you may have and portray a self-confident image.

Using a Low Tone

It doesn't matter whether you are male or female, if you are nervous or lacking self-confidence, it has a way of showing in your voice. I am not talking about having a shaky voice; what I am referring to is the fast-talking pace and high pitches associated with nervous people.

If you must mask your anxiety and nervousness, you must learn how to work on your tone of voice. Decreasing the pace with which you speak and lowering your tone will convey more self-confidence and even power.

To lower your voice tone to its optimal level, use this trick. Tighten your lips for about 10 to 15 seconds while you hum. Obviously, you should do this in private before you start talking to others.

Here's something else that can convey confidence in your tone: let your voice drop when you finish off your sentences to give them more power. A high pitch at the end of your sentences makes it sound as if you are asking a question or seeking approval from your listeners. In a speech, there is something known as the "authoritative arc." Here's a brief summary of how that works. When you speak, let your voice start from one tone, and then slightly raise the pitch in the middle of your sentence, and finally drop the pitch to a low tone as you finish off your sentence. Practice this for a while and you'll get really good at it.

Assume the Power Pose

Stand upright, legs apart, hands on your hips, and hold your head high like a confident person. This is known as the power pose. It is one of the instances where your brain releases hormones that increase your confidence level and reduce your stress level simply by changing your body posture. When you assume this pose for about 3 minutes, it makes you calmer and more confident. This is particularly helpful if you are anxious about a meeting you have to attend.

Conclusion

I began the first chapter of this book with a bold assertion: *we lie a lot!* This doesn't necessarily mean that we intend to hurt others. In fact, sometimes – if not most times – the reason we lie is to protect others, especially those we love. But when I said that we lie a lot, I did not only mean lying verbally. As a matter of fact, the lies we tell non-verbally seem to outweigh those we tell verbally. I have taken the time to carefully show you how you can easily correlate these two – the verbal and non-verbal communications.

My goal for writing this book is to help you and every other person who seek to improve their interpersonal relationships. We are social beings who are bound to interact with others who make up our personal and professional world. Since communicating with others is not limited to only words, there is a need to have a thorough understanding of other forms of human communication so that our interactions can become richer, fuller, and more meaningful.

There are countless schools that teach us how to read and write words right from when we are old enough to speak. However, there is a scarcity of formal schools that teach us how to read and decode body language. To fill this yearning gap, I have written this book using easy-to-understand terms so that anyone can read, understand, and apply the tips, tricks, and techniques.

If there is one message I would like to leave you with, it is that there is no static meaning to a particular body language. This is why it is very important to first and foremost develop your people-reading skills. This will help you to form a baseline behavior for the people who are a big part of your life so that you can properly decode their non-verbal intent with a greater degree of accuracy.

After reading this book, you may be tempted to rush into giving meaning to every single body movement you observe. Resist that temptation. It is not necessary to immediately start interpreting what everyone is saying with their body language. What is important right now is for you to start building your observational ability. I urge you to follow the tips given in chapter 1 to help you achieve this very important first step.

Equally, it is important to start working on your non-verbal cues. What are the messages you would like others to receive from you? What do you want your handshake to convey in a particular setting? How do you want others to begin to perceive you? Take the time to practice and develop the necessary gestures, facial expressions, body postures, and body movements that convey exactly what you want. If you do not already know how to do this, the chapter on how to fake your body language will come in handy.

There are times when you will not readily have what it takes to make a good impression due to anxiety or outright fear of the situation. Sometimes it could be because you have not yet mastered how to summon at will the desired body language you need to convey the right message. In such cases, you will need to *"fake it till you make it."*

Always remember that not very many people are trained in the art of deception, therefore, their words are likely not to correlate with their body language when they attempt to be deceptive. This will not be obvious if you do not know how to read their non-verbal cues. So, give all you can to mastering the techniques outlined in this book and you will become great at pinpointing when others try to mask their true intention with words that say something else.

However, I would like to caution against interacting with people with the notion that everyone you meet is trying to deceive you or hide their intention from you. That will make you live a paranoid and mistrusting kind of life. Give yourself a break from trying to figure out everyone's true intentions. Allow people to live their lives just as you should focus on living and improving yours.

Don't ever substitute enjoying the moments you share with the people in your life for a life of unfounded suspicion. Always keep this principle in mind and let it guide you: if there is nothing at stake in a situation or in an interaction, ignore the urge to try to read every single body cue of everyone involved in the interaction. The knowledge contained in this book should be used only when the need arises. And believe me, the need doesn't arise as frequently as you think it does. Even though body language abounds in almost every interaction and communication, it is not necessary to read every single sign because they, more often than not, are not conveying anything significantly different than the words being spoken in the communication.

Finally, I strongly recommend that you read and study this book more than once. Do not forget to put into practice what you read. It is only in the practical application that you can gain mastery. You may not become an expert at reading people. In fact, reading body language is not an exact science to begin with. Nevertheless, you will definitely get good at it to the point where you can use it to improve your current relationships and interactions.

CPSIA information can be obtained
at www.ICGtesting.com
Printed in the USA
LVHW052220100221
678887LV00009B/272

9 781801 686938